'Insights Into Pain & Suffering'

A guide to Neuropathic Pain and Complex Regional Pain
Syndrome, known as Reflex Sympathetic Dystrophy

'David R Blake,
Jenny Lewis, Candy McCabe
and Catherine Taylor'

ISBN: 1-905553-14-5

Printed for
BookPrintingWorld
www.bookprintingworld.com
in the UK

Professor David R Blake FRCP

Professor Blake is a consultant Rheumatologist with a longstanding clinical and scientific interest in pain and inflammation. He has published widely in these areas. He was awarded the Heberden Medal by The British Society for Rheumatology for his contributions to research in these areas.

He leads a clinical research group at the Royal National Hospital for Rheumatic Diseases Bath UK and is the professor of Locomotor Sciences at the University of Bath UK.

David Blake is patron of RSD UK.

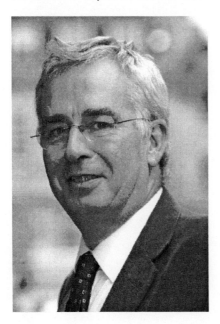

Professor Dame Carol Black; DBE PRCP FMed Sci

"Modern medicine is about partnership-partnership between patients, their doctors and all the many other health professionals whose experience, understanding and skills may be sought when we are ill. This unusual book explores partnership through dialogue.

The narratives gathered from scores of people with this strange, bewildering and distressing pain syndrome bring a challenge to medical science; but they also call us to recognise, confront and overcome ignorance of unexplained clinical phenomena, and to beware of hasty and sometimes heartless judgements about a cruel, isolating and often intractable kind of suffering.

In the instances presented here are frank, sensitive, thoughtful, listening explorations of the poorly understood, often unrecognised, and frequently misjudged problems that are the subject of this book. The narratives are a humbling challenge to our understanding and to our caring.

The book reminds us too that among our tasks as physicians is to interpret the problems that patients bring, with sensitivity, imagination, and a humane curiosity matched by humility." Royal College of Physicians, London UK.

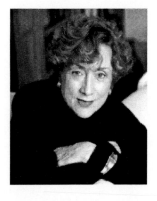

12th March 2006

2

Preface

A book for patients, carers, doctors, lawyers and students of pain

Many people have contributed to this book. These include members of RSD UK with CRPS, their families and carers, CRPS patients who attend the Royal National Hospital for Rheumatic Diseases in Bath (UK), and the clinical, educational and research group that supports them.

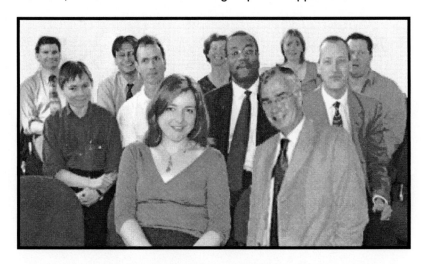

Here are some of the latter, a great bunch of enthusiasts
with big brains and larger hearts

Judith Beresford-Smith, Sheila Blake, Helen Cohen, Jonathan Cole, Lucy Cory, Carol Dyer, Sandy Derham, Iain Dorrington, David Elvins, Rachel Edwards, Richard Gregory, Richard Haigh, Jane Hall, Nigel Harris, Simon Harrison, Peter Hollingworth, William House, Helen Jerina, Keri Johnson, Alison MacKenzie, Edward Keogh, Cathy Richards, Karen Rodham, Rachel Morris, Julie Rowlinson, Nick Shenker, Cliff Stevens, Barry Taylor Amanda Thompson, Sin-Ti Towlson, Dianne Venn, and Adrian Williams.

Thanks. March 1 2006

It is our dream…

…that this book will be used as a basis for discussion; not only by patients and their carers, but also by those who train students in medicine, the law and associated disciplines.

"Understanding is curing ignorance and curing ignorance is abolishing fear".

Matt Marty

"Alice was beginning to get very tired of sitting by her sister on the bank, and of having nothing to do: once or twice she had peeped into the book her sister was reading, but it had no pictures or conversations in it, "and what is the use of a book," thought Alice, "without pictures or conversations?"

Lewis Carol

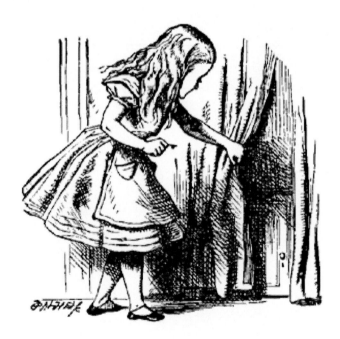

It has been written...

...in a clear type script with hefty gaps for the simple reason that patients with CRPS/RSD find concentration difficult. For many the letters will shimmer and sometimes move, or read 'odd', like 'ddo', which is distressing, but explainable. Many pictures are included as one of our patients said; "I only read books with pictures, David" and so we put them in just for *Rosy*.

It is written in two parts. The first is based upon patient dialogues, narratives, and their interpretation. The second part is a fully referenced scientific review.

The first is written in standard prose and rarely referenced to aid digestion; the second using the language of the scientific literature.

We are grateful...

...to members of RSD UK who helped us write this book. We are appreciative of the tolerance shown by many other sufferers, with severe disease, we have met whilst struggling to understand this disease. They have by their openness, helped us understand some of the mechanisms that drive 'the pain network' in the brain that underpins this syndrome. This is an illness that may be very mild, but occasionally catastrophic, and often far worse than the injury that started it. As with all chronic illnesses recovery requires you to be informed, patient and proactive.

We acknowledge with thanks the support we have received from the Arthritis Research Campaign (UK), and the Dipex Organisation which taught us the importance of patient experiences as an aid to understanding. The Gwen Bush Foundation helped us initiate many pilot studies along the road.

We pay tribute to Gwen Bush, who though having spent many years of her life in pain, lost neither the courage to go on nor her concern for others.

Table of contents: Part 1

9

A few words of introduction

Where we tell you who this book is for, why we wrote it and why we chose an unusual style of delivery. We show some of the other names for this syndrome. We mention how important early treatment is for a good and fast recovery, though it is never too late to start. We describe, through narrative and dialogue, the severe pain known as allodynia and the words used to describe the many pains of CRPS and some of the emotions that develop. We demonstrate certain simple images that can worsen pain and caution those that are easily stimulated by visual images.

We consider common symptoms first – pains
The most common symptom allodynia is explained more fully in the context of many other pains.

The symptoms and signs of neurogenic inflammation
We describe some of the basic clinical signs and symptoms and depict these with a few pictures, tell you about inflammation and describe neurogenic inflammation.

What is Complex Regional Pain Syndrome?
The question posed here is how do we classify this disease? We introduce taxonomy and demystify how a diagnosis is established and point out some of the difficulties. We introduce and describe factor analysis and why you want to know about it even though you may have never heard of it.

More clinical pictures
Armed with this knowledge we introduce more clinical pictures and link them to factor analysis. Now you are getting the knowledge.

What causes CRPS?
The range of serious injuries is presented and linked to many trivial ones. The sufferer wonders, why me and why these and why now?
Making a diagnosis; laboratory tests
The tests we have available to help diagnose CRPS and exclude other problems is described. The strengths and weaknesses of the tests are discussed in terms of sensitivity and specificity.

The concept of central pain
The nervous system both peripheral and central is described, myths and prejudice exposed and the concept of networks introduced. Clever stuff, but well worth knowing.

Moving on with more dialogues and stories
We link pain and emotion and talk of rejection, anger and depression.

Spreading CRPS and telling us about connections in the network
We talk of CRPS that spreads to the bowel, bladder and genitalia.
We discuss CRPS that is confined to the bowel or bladder. We talk dirty, discussing through dialogues, sex, penetration, stimulation and orgasms since most books don't and it matters.

Phantoms, pain and swelling
Here we tackle strange symptoms that are common, distressing and rarely discussed. Things like phantoms, apparitions, ghouls and ghosts and draw comparisons with amputation pain.

Treatment and beyond
As we move towards a scientific analysis of CRPS we describe, in a light-hearted way, how to behave in a clinic and what to expect. Inappropriate underclothes for women are illustrated for the benefit of our younger male readers.

We move slowly towards treatment and introduce many practical problems caused by CRPS and the perceptual difficulties they cause. We extend, in increments, scientific knowledge suggesting the importance of the brain as the central source of CRPS and indicate which bits do what and what goes awry.

How to get things better as quickly as possible
With this knowledge we describe a screening questionnaire that assists with the rehabilitation programme. This is described in detail.

Drugs, but don't hold your breath
The title speaks for itself, but we describe opiates, anticonvulsants antidepressants, antiarrhyhmics, blocking the sympathetic system, spinal cord simulation, and hyperbaric oxygen and more.

A few words on genetics and inheritance
We discuss what genetics is all about and how far we have come and what needs to be done; which is a lot.

Does CRPS have a purpose?
Sounds like a daft question, but biology is based on purpose and without an understanding of what the benefits of CRPS could be in an evolutionary sense we will never understand this disease fully.

Much more to say, but time to stop
A few summary remarks take us to RSD UK, the charity, written by Ms Catherine Taylor, the woman who started it all and who inspired this book. Then, a moving poem followed by a final story about allodynia that is personal to DRB, who compiled this classic.

The Epilogue
...is about "stories and story telling". A personal tale or narrative of allodynia and the response of individuals, family, friends, doctors, lawyers and a dead body

Useful reading and web sites

And part 2- A scientific review

For those who want to know more and who wrote what of importance

IMPORTANT NOTE

Sufferers diagnosed and treated early usually do very well with medical intervention. Those who have developed a persistent disease have contributed their stories for the benefit of others and in the hope that it will improve both medical and public awareness of this condition.

The book, therefore, does not accurately reflect the experience of the many CRPS patients, detected early and treated promptly, who don't have much of a story to tell and don't tell it.

PART 1

CRPS: Stories, dialogues and thoughts

The worst pain imaginable, allodynia in CRPS
[Fig 1 pg i]

Pain is no evil unless it conquers us.
George Eliot

"I was assured by everyone that the sharp, burning, excruciating pain in my leg would be OK with rest, but OK never came. Instead it felt as if my leg had been doused in gasoline and set on fire. I suffered constant muscle spasm, my leg became swollen, sweated profusely, and was cold." This is a quote from the Web.

This little book describes the most painful of all recognised chronic human pain conditions, CRPS/RSD. It has been compiled from narratives and dialogues of sufferers whose diagnosis was delayed. It is a book about pain, suffering, anger, rejection, betrayal and fortitude.

CRPS, also known as RSD.

[Figs 2 & 3 pages i, ii]

"I was told by a health professional that RSD is a fancy name for being lazy and not using a Limb."

(A mother of an 11-year-old child with RSD.)

The authors try to explain this occasionally intractable condition. We hope it is of help to the many who endure this disease and those who support them.

The problem

13

"I had to deal with more pain than I had ever felt before but nobody knew what was wrong with me. I got sent to loads of different kinds of doctors. Every time I got prodded and poked and pulled around, this was extremely painful. They always stabbed in the same places and then asked all the same questions. Then they told me they couldn't find anything wrong. I was so confused and sometimes it felt like I was going mad and that nobody believed me. It took 11 months before a doctor diagnosed RSD." It takes many more a lot longer.

"Just how many diseases have I got, doc?"

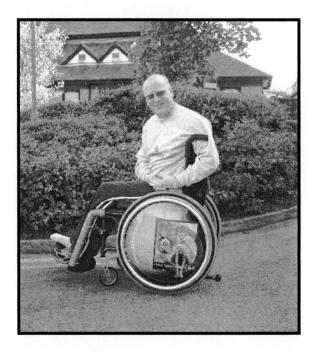

At the RSD UK conference - a designer wheel

Oh, what a muddle. Many names have been given to this disease including Complex Regional Pain Syndrome, Algodystrophy, Reflex Sympathetic Dystrophy, Variable Pain Syndrome, Sudeck's dystrophy and Causalgia.

And so to the language of pain

"The quality of our thoughts is bordered on all sides by our facility with language."

J. Michael Straczynski.

Pain is a "**perception**" which we communicate "as thoughts and feelings, through a system of signals, such as voice-sounds and gestures". Let us analyse this sentence first because it is crucial to understanding the dialogues and stories we present.

What do we mean by 'sensation' and 'perception'? And what's the big deal about the difference?

We take in information, lots of it, via our senses. Our brains interpret it as a 'percept' which is something perceived by our senses. For instance we take in visual information as different wavelengths of light and convert it into colour, shape and texture. The eyes sense but the brain sees. Each individual prioritises, so we may all receive a similar visual stimulus and perceive it very differently.

> "It is the mind which creates the world around us, and even though we stand side by side in the same meadow, my eyes will never see what is beheld by yours, my heart will never stir to the emotions with which yours is touched."
>
> George Gissing 1857-1903

Pain is no different; we receive an injurious stimulus to our nerves, we sense its dangerous qualities and we interpret that in a variety of ways. We interpret injury as multiple 'percepts', by our senses. Pain is one of these percepts.

Pain is not really a sensation it is a perception. We all differ in our responses to simple sensory inputs, both from each other, and from other species. Therefore there is no reason to believe that we interpret dangerous stimuli in the same or identical fashion. There are profound similarities of course, but great differences.

Many factors influence pain perception, genetics being one, previous exposure to painful stimuli another. Racial, cultural and other factors all play a part. The importance of any one varies with circumstance. There are therefore near-infinite pain perceptions, but the sufferer and outsider tolerates and understands some more than others. This is a quote obtained from the RSD UK web site.

"My leg feels like it is going to be sick. My leg is killing me."
Jenna, a young girl with CRPS.

Pain also creates reflex behaviours that are less controllable. The withdrawal of the injured hand from the fire, the grimace and the spontaneous speech are the most obvious. These have a defensive purpose, in warning others who may be about to stray into danger and importantly to gain attention and to attract help.

Pain is generally an unpleasant and unwelcome perception, but there are exceptions when it is used to enhance sexual pleasure. Pain is linked to many primitive emotional centres in the brain; anger is one. The vocal language of pain depicts this and tells us something about strongly activated brain networks. Let us consider a spectrum of words used to describe pain. In this book certain words cluster together and are much less commonly used in other painful states. Different languages use different words with different meanings though the principles are similar.

Words you may use

Commonly used words include sharp, stabbing, gnawing, tingling, burning, fiery, piercing, prickly and lancing. Others might include excruciating, agonising, smouldering, loathsome, intolerable, foul, disgusting, raw, hateful, agonising, unbearable, detestable, repugnant, odious, obnoxious and spiteful.

The language used by health professionals and scientists is briefer, but unfathomable to any one other than a specialist.

16

Pain can be 'acute' or 'chronic'. It can embrace 'hyperaesthesia, hyperalgesia and allodynia' or it may link to a cause such as neuropathic, which is nerve injury. This book deals with people who have 'hyperaesthesia, hyperalgesia and allodynia'. Sometimes the cause is 'neuropathic'. We describe these words fully as they matter to those who assess you for medical, legal or benefit related reasons. You may call your pain 'disgusting', the professionals will not. Indeed, it may have a negative connotation to the least informed of them.

Hyperaesthesia

"That pin felt really sharp," is an example of **hyperaesthesia**.

She responded in an exaggerated way to a mild pin prick is an example of hyperalgesia. The first, hyperaesthesia, is a symptom; the second, hyperalgesia, is a physical sign. It describes an amplified response to a painful stimulus. A sensory input creates an exaggerated perceptual output.

Allodynia

"That touch was painful." is an example of **allodynia**. This is a big difference from hyperaesthesia.
Allodynia is pain experienced from a non-painful stimulus such as touch or even sound. The pain may be felt a long way from the injured part. This time an innocuous sensory input produces an extreme perceptual output.

Allodynia can occur after nerve injury or without nerve injury. In the first case it is called 'neuropathic'. As we know more and more about the zillions of fine nerves in our skin, and how they signal, we appreciate that all injuries create a degree of nerve damage. The separation is therefore, we suggest, rather artificial.

Allodynic pain, with its expanded perceptual outputs suggests that the 'focus of control' has spread to the 'central nervous system' or CNS. We believe it to be outside the control of the injured part. We come back to this again and again after we have read the stories and the recorded dialogues. The key medical-scientific question, we are nudging towards is; is CRPS is a 'central pain syndrome'?

This book is about people with allodynic pain who have developed this condition in response to an injury, albeit sometimes trivial. The perceptual pain response is out of the control of the peripheral sensory system and in the hands of the CNS. We describe the symptoms and signs and 'have a go' at an explanation.

The explanation is not complete as our understanding of the science of CRPS has a way to go. However we know enough to suggest treatment programmes that should reset the dysfunctional 'painstat' (compare 'thermostat') which is where, it seems, the problem lies. Where is this device that automatically responds to sensory changes and activates switches to control both the perceptual output and the reflex reactions that characterise CRPS?

The perceptual outputs are symptoms, the reflex reactions in the periphery are clinical signs. Analysing and interpreting symptoms and signs correctly is the job of health professionals. Medical-legal lawyers take action against us, on behalf of patients if we fail and that failure is thought unreasonable.

This is not an easy disease to have and it is often hard to analyse. We will take it in steps. The book is written on an educational model of repetition, but at each cycle we add a little more detail.

The salesman's tale

**Tell 'em what you are going to tell 'em.
Tell 'em.
Tell 'em what you told 'em.**

Your symptoms as stories and dialogues

Pain is a very common symptom of CRPS, but may not be invariable throughout the course of the disease. Here are some descriptions of 'the pains' which accompany the many signs that help characterise CRPS.

"My knee joint feels like a red hot poker you put in between the joint then continuously moved up and down. My skin feels like when you get bad sunburn, all you need is a little tiny knock and it feels like somebody's whacked you".

"My arm is like a burning, aching sensation. The fingers feel stiff sometimes; I think because of the coldness they feel stiff. I would say sometimes it's definitely a nerve pain because you can't seem to get rid of it with any sort of pain killer, analgesia".

"It's that painful that you can't sit down, you've got to sort of keep walking about and everything all the time because it's very irritating. There's not one thing I've found that, when I'm in a lot of pain will ease that pain and I've just got to be up and about walking around and pacing and it's frustrating and it really, gets on top of you"

"I mean, I think the pain and everything that I have with this condition is certainly a lot worse than anything that I've had before in my entire life. Nothing at all compares ...by then I had a job to watch the television; you had a job to concentrate on anything because now from... scoring say four or five during the day this, this poker sensation that was off a scale of ten. During the course of the evening it began to get worse."

"I was lying in bed and... it literally felt as if somebody had put a tourniquet at the top of my arm... and it was like a bicycle pump and they were, literally blowing my arm up. And when it got to that stage my arm was just going to explode."

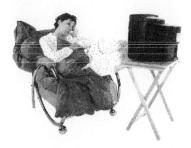

A story

"July 16th 1997 will always be burned in my mind. It was the day my life ended. I arrived at hospital for a carpal tunnel operation (CTS) to my hand." [Fig.4 page ii]

"The consultant came to see me, explained about the procedure. He told me this is the first time he had performed CTS on someone who was awake. I didn't realise I was going to be awake, that came as a shock."

I was wheeled down to theatre when the bloke first put the tourniquet on. I said that you can only have it on for so long and he agreed. I always thought it was 20-30 minutes. I was watching the clock all the time and kept saying the tourniquet has to come off soon! And they kept saying won't be long now! It was on for over an hour.

I was discharged a couple of hours later. Mum and Dad picked me up. The hour drive was awful. I felt all the bumps and was in pain. My hand really hurt. By the evening I couldn't understand why my hand was hurting so much. I took pain killers; they were useless."
"The next couple of day's things didn't improve. My hand felt as if it was on fire, it was so hot, and the pain awful. Anyway I thought it will soon settle down. Just bite a pillow and take another pain killer. I never let the kids see me shed a tear. It was hard not to dress James or change his nappies."

"When the consultant removed my bandages, the hand was in a strange position, what I can only described as a hook. The fingers were all together and my thumb was in a very strange position too. I later renamed my hand 'the claw'. The skin was red and shiny, and the temperature was so hot. I could not move fingers or wrist. When the nurse wanted me to open my hand and twist my wrist to remove the stitches it was not an easy feat. When she touched my hand I nearly hit the roof. They looked at me as if I was a naughty child. I was scared and frightened."

"I could not understand what was wrong with my hand, why my fingers wouldn't open. I was told they would be ok; just use them."

"The bus journey home was hell. I felt every movement, wind was hurting me, my hand was throbbing, and burning and I was finding it so hard not to cry. I couldn't give the bus driver the money; he had to open my purse. I felt so scared."

Another story

Whilst there are differences, we present this so that the similarities in presentation of hyperalgesia and allodynia are obvious. The words and the emotional responses are the key clues.

"I fell and landed on my right hand side. I heard a snap followed by an intense pain in the left side of my left foot. I saw the doctor who checked the x rays and confirmed that there was no break. Perhaps the ligaments were ripped, but there was no way that they could tell and to leave it for a week. If it still hurt then I was to return."

"A nurse bandaged it up and I was offered crutches. A week later my foot was still very painful. On attending my next appointment they confirmed that there are no broken bones and the specialist suggests that it is a tendon injury, and the leg should be plastered for three weeks. The foot remained sore and a throbbing sensation was felt most of the time."

So far both stories tell of an insult. The first describes a common enough problem, a trapped nerve in the wrist and the second a nasty fall. In the first case you may, as we did, think that this lady had an amplified pain response already, she was fearful and intolerant of the tourniquet. The second sounds like a significant ligamentous tear. In both cases rest and immobilization are unhelpful and things are getting worse. The allodynia is now obvious from the descriptions. However, in both cases, the problem might be that there is still substantial injury and time will cure. If this is wrong, it is a serious mistake. The immediate treatment for acute CRPS is the opposite: Movement. Let us return to the story. "On returning to have the plaster removed the foot was looked at. The specialist seeing that it was still very swollen and painful to the touch suggested that it should be re-plastered for four weeks; this time only to use the leg very occasionally, and to keep it elevated at all times where possible."

"A little later I was walking from the lounge to the kitchen when I felt a very sharp pain in the left foot and almost a burning sensation again, I thought that this might settle. It did not and I attended the Accident and Emergency department. They suggested the plaster was removed again. The foot was still swollen, and this was two months after the accident. A plaster was put back but the front was left open allowing the leg to swell."

"On starting physiotherapy I could only walk with an eggshell weight on my foot, and they got me exercising my foot and ankle in numerous ways. Getting in and out of the bath at this time was a near impossibility.

"I made an appointment to see my doctor. I was very depressed and burst into tears and told her that I am finding it very hard to cope with the mundane things in life and being trapped in my own house. Work rang me to say that if I did not return back to work before the twelve months was up they would terminate my employment."

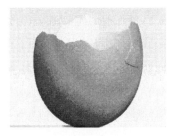

Unable to bear touch and nerves cracking and ragged.
[www.rebecca.hitherby.com]

"A specialist pain consultant has recommended acupuncture… when the needles are placed in my normal leg lumps have appeared"

"At present I feel frustrated and upset that no one seems to be able to help me. My love life is non-existent… even bedding touching me hurts...please help me."

22

These are two common enough injuries, but the responses are not. They have been a personal and family tragedy. These are unusual response to injuries and few doctors see many cases in a working lifetime.

The allodynic features are not being recognized, the diagnosis is not made and appropriate treatment is being delayed. Success in treating this disease comes when the diagnosis is made promptly and sophisticated exercise programmes delivered with the support of specially trained professional staff.

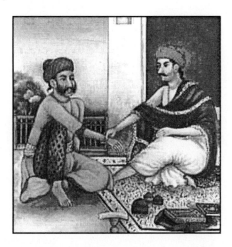

Matching symptoms and signs to make a diagnosis is not easy, particularly in the early stages when treatment is needed urgently.

One way of picking up early allodynia is to ask two questions.
Is the pain superficial or deep?
Does it have a burning quality?
Allodynic pain is "deep burning" and often described in emotive words.
If it develops inside a fracture cast the part feels far too tight.

We will return to symptoms throughout the book, but now to a few clinical signs. We have heard of a few in the stories already.

Neurogenic inflammation

The signs relate to a form of inflammation that develops in this syndrome, called neurogenic inflammation. This describes an inflammatory reaction, not caused by trauma or damage necessarily, but by discharging nerves.

Inflammation is associated with 'cardinal signs and symptoms' described first by the ancient Greeks and in particular Galen. Cardinal here, meaning basic, central and important.

The cardinal symptoms and signs of inflammation

Redness, heat, swelling and loss of function are signs and then there are two symptoms, pain and heat. Heat is a physical sign the investigator can feel and also a symptom, a feeling or percept. Wherever inflammation occurs these signs are present to a variable extent, but CRPS throws up some others because of the very powerful and unusual nerve discharges.

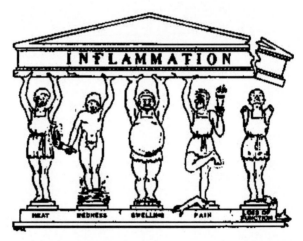

From the archives of the late Prof. D. Willoughby, London.

"...the hand was in a _strange position_, what I can only describe as a hook."

"The skin was _red and shiny_" and "the temperature was so _hot_ and I could _not move_ my fingers or wrist."

"It (my foot) was _swollen_ and the _nails grow_ long and are _brittle_ and it _sweats_ on its own."

"When the needles are placed in my normal leg, _lumps_ have appeared."

Neurogenic inflammation can be seen on Fig 5 page iii.

Classical early CRPS is often easy to reverse with repeated desensitisation and graded exercises.

The foot is a dusky blue, the foot and lower leg are swollen, the skin beads with perspiration and the nails are starting to deform. The foot is turning in.

These symptoms and signs seem quite distinctive. As you will see from the colour pictures that follow, they can be very variable. Do they make a precise medical diagnosis?

What is Complex Regional Pain Syndrome?

So far we have described, through patients' voices, the pain and suffering that comes with bad disease. Not everybody, by a long way, has all these symptoms; much more often they are less severe and only of short duration.

Some of the basic characteristics, nevertheless, are found in most including strange pains, frustration, anxiety and bewilderment. Most will have variable colour changes, swelling and sweating around the painful area at some time.

How do we classify this disease?

Taxonomy is a word derived from the Greek. The medical profession like Greek and Latin derived words as they make us appear clever and justify a large cheque in the private sector. Taxonomy is simply a way of categorising things.

It means the cataloguing or sorting of biological stuff, such as organisms or diseases. You classify, you sub-classify and you split sub-classifications into different bits, and so on. Classifications are not fixed and often change as knowledge grows. Sometimes they prove wrong.

Here is taxonomy. Neuropathic pain, or the pain of nerve injury, might be a starting point, allodynia falls within it. CRPS is an example of allodynia and splits again into two types CRPS 1 and CRPS 2, which we dissect later.

CRPS is a disease or disorder of merged symptoms and signs, following different kinds of trauma. It has different causes and outcomes. The outcomes range from trivial which is the usual, to very severe which is much rarer. It is referred to as a syndrome to illustrate to doctors that it is diagnosed by the pattern of a set of symptoms and signs. It is none the less a disease, sometimes mild but occasionally dreadful.

Making a simple taxonomy

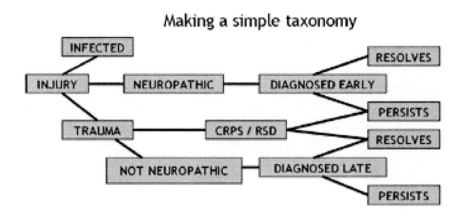

CRPS types

CRPS types 1 and 2, are defined by the 'International Association for the Study of Pain' following a 'multiaxial factor analysis and classification of chronic pains'. This is a fancy way of describing a difficult scientific analysis conducted by doctors and scientists with experience. The trick is to be referred to one. This is not easy if neither you nor your doctor have the first idea what is the matter.

"...I've been all round the country; I've been to see numerous specialists all round the country and not one of them could actually tell me that, what was actually wrong with me."

"Yes my diagnosis was slow, easily five years of waiting and wanting to know what's wrong with you... it was a great relief finding out what was wrong. A huge weight lifted off my shoulders knowing that somebody actually knows what's wrong with me. I mean, it was just so comforting finding out that you're not stupid and you're not like making things up and that there are other people that's had to suffer the same things that I have."

It is unclear how common CRPS is as it may occur in many forms. What figures do exist suggest that around one to two percent of people will get CRPS after a ligamentous injury to the wrist and many more after a fracture. Indeed up to thirty-five per cent will get a small degree of allodynia and temperature change. Around five per cent will get it after a nerve injury. It occurs in roughly one percent of people who have had a stroke.

We estimate, without good figures, that the incidence of chronic problems that exemplify this book are around two per cent of the acute population. The reason this figure is nothing more than a guess, is that where it is studied carefully knowledge is by definition good, and treatment prompt.

There are 1,800 members most with CRPS registered with RSD UK; which must be a small fraction of the total, but may be is representative of the worst cases. Of course, in order to know how common something is, you need to know what it is you are describing and that is difficult in many diseases and near impossible in some.

Here is taxonomy of CRPS derived in 1995, and it separates the disease in to two subsets.

CRPS Type 1 is also known as Reflex Sympathetic Dystrophy (RSD)
Type 1 is a syndrome that develops after an initiating noxious event.

Spontaneous pain or allodynia/hyperalgesia occurs that is not limited to the territory of a single peripheral nerve and is disproportionate to the initiating event.
There is or has been evidence of oedema (swelling), skin blood flow abnormality (colour and temperature) or abnormal sudomotor (sweating) activity in the region of the pain since the initiating event.

This diagnosis is excluded by the existence of conditions that may account for the degree of pain and dysfunction.

CRPS Type 2 is a syndrome that develops after a nerve injury; otherwise it is the same as type 1. The distinction is a little artificial, as all injuries create nerve injury at a microscopic level.

Modified criteria have been proposed for research studies. They are more detailed and identify motor abnormalities such as tremor, trembling and altered movements of an automatic nature.

We mentioned previously, and without elaboration, that these criteria were determined by 'factor analyses'. Let us expand; it will help to explain why some symptoms cluster together and why some may occur without others.

Not all CRPS sufferers look the same

Some people get immense pain that dominates. Some do not, but may have dramatic temperature changes and see large changes in the colour of their limbs. Others may do either, neither or both, but swell with oedema fluid and 'sweat buckets'.

CRPS patients may have very different symptoms and signs. Some look completely normal at first glance – Figs.6, 7, 8 pg iii, iv.

Often there are dramatic differences between CRPS subjects. One group has hands or feet that hurt variably, but finds it difficult to move. They may shake or have involuntary movements. This subset often has 'trophic symptoms and signs'. For instance, clawing of the hands is common and they may clench them involuntarily. Feet may turn in, with the soles of the feet looking not downwards but inwards. There may be toe and fingernail growth that is excessive and different from the other side.

Factor analysis has been defined as 'a statistical technique that identifies coherent, and conceptually linked, subsets of variables within a data set'. To put it another way, it's a way of sub-classifying. For instance some of us will get cancer, but is it benign or malignant? Is it isolated or widespread? What is its prognostic sub-classification, based on a microscopic analysis?

We assume that since some signs and symptoms link together they share a similar underlying or connecting stimulus that drives them. That is one of the purposes of undertaking a factor analysis; to establish if there is a central control point or determine if there is more than one. Another definition is this:

'Factor analysis' examines the pattern of inter-connections between symptoms and signs, known as variables. The technique determines whether there are subsets of variables called factors which associate highly with each other, but that show a poor relationship with other or factors. Or to say it more simply, "do some symptoms always come with others, but not necessarily with them all?"

We list the 'factors' together as best we can.

Factor [A]
Allodynia signs. Allodynia symptoms.

Remember hyperalgesia is an excessive pain response to a painful stimulus. Allodynia is a pain response to a non-painful stimulus.

Factor [B]
Temperature differences between limbs. Temperature symptoms. Colour change signs.

Factor [C]
Oedema signs. Oedema symptoms.
Sweating differences between the limbs.

Factor [D]
Decreased range of motion signs.
Decreased range of motion symptoms.
Motor dysfunction signs.
Motor dysfunction symptoms, trophic symptoms.
Trophic signs.

The symptoms and signs in each group link with each other but don't link that closely with the other factors.

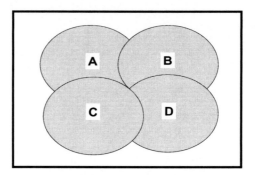

Factors A, B, C and D linking a little to create 'full-blown' CRPS

How factor analysis helps scientists but confuses doctors and lawyers

Let us discuss a case described to one of us.

"Professor, I am so pleased to see you and your team," says Mr. Townsend.
"Good morning."

"I understand from the RSD-UK website that you claim to be an expert in whatever disease I have: CRPS, RSD, Soo-Decks something…"

I smile thinking about the downside of changing nomenclature based on ill-considered taxonomies.

"Well not exactly, as you know being a Web man all these diseases are the same. The disease has been called many names over the years: Causalgia, Sudeck's Dystrophy, Reflex Sympathetic Dystrophy or RSD and others."

"Good, look at the hand, it's horrible, the pain is disgusting and it's stiffening up. The problem is it doesn't swell…well it does, but you can't see it." He explains with growing frustration.

"Take your time, no rush."

"What do you mean - the problem is that it isn't swollen?"

"Well", he says," its two problems really. My wife says, because she can't see it swelling that I'm exaggerating … and the lawyers and doctors for the other side say it doesn't meet the 'criteria for RSD".

"May I examine you?" I respond, "I will not need to touch you, no worries. Please look at my sign."

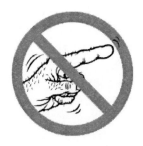

"No touching in this clinic"

From: www.creativebits.org/ taxonomy/creativeego

He examines himself. I watch as he points out the distribution of his pain symptoms. I observe how he responds to his own light touch, how he responds to touching himself, with a warm tube, with cotton wool, and with a needle.

I give him my hand and ask him to touch himself with it as lightly as he touched himself. I ask him to explain the differences in these feelings. I ask him about swelling, its distribution and where it feels swollen. I ask how the symptoms change when he closes his eyes.

I look at the pattern of sweating and the colour.

"I'm almost done," I explain. A few tests with the team and we will dictate a report for your doctor, in front of you."
This man has classical CRPS. His full history had not suggested alternative pathologies. His injury, a blow by a porter when collecting second-hand furniture, caused no fracture or obvious nerve injury.

However, the initial trauma was at a place of work. He has now developed CRPS type 1, with factor clustering in subsets A and D. Slight asymmetric sweating suggests partial factor C development and true swelling may develop later. His 'phantom' swelling is, we believe, part of a Factor A grouping, linking with the allodynic pain component.

Lawyers, like doctors, vary in their knowledge of CRPS/RSD. Here is a story told by a lawyer with CRPS. It is taken from his web page. It describes the difference between law and justice.

> "In my first year of law school, my contracts professor 'set up' [tricked] a fellow student. Proper application of the law in accordance with the facts of the case resulted in a horrendous and unjust ruling. When the professor asked how the student felt about the court's conclusion, she said she understood that this was a proper application of the law; but the result was unfair. The professor nearly went berserk. He shouted, "Fair? Young lady, the law is the law and justice is justice; and if you want justice, go across the street!" and he pointed toward the divinity school where future priests were taught."

A bad joke, as old as the hills

"Counsellor, you should be aware that at this point, what you are saying is just going in one ear and out the other."
"Your honour," replied the lawyer, "That goes without saying. What is there to prevent it?"

A medical legal story and a poem from a colleague, a consultant rheumatologist.

"CRPS triggered by injury often comes to litigation. I thought I was wise to the difficulties in preparing medical reports for these claimants but I still get caught out.

The principal difficulty is convincing the lawyers about CRPS. Here we have a story of a minor injury triggering pain in, say, a hand that is so severe it is impossible to use, it is so sensitive that even a breeze hurts it, it stops someone even dressing, it goes on for months and the doctors aren't getting it better. This defies everyday human experience. I must firstly convince the lawyers the condition actually exists and secondly it is as severe as the patients describe. This is difficult enough even where there are barn-door signs of temperature and colour changes. But when the signs are subtle or absent, even the patients are confused about the condition, let alone the lawyers.

With this in mind, I include the let-out clause 'another's pain is unknowable; the only way the claimant can be shown to be misleading is if they are observed performing an action they say they can never perform, even on their best day'. This is code for 'covert surveillance', a tidy industry of usually ex-policemen with hidden video cameras following the claimant for a day or two: I am then presented with the recording.

Usually the recording confirms the account the claimant gave of what they could and could not do. Occasionally, I realise that I have been duped. But Miss T had me stumped.

I believed Miss T, she complained of severe pain in her right hand, she could never use it normally and she certainly couldn't consider using it to turn a door key or carry shopping. The physical signs were few and the lawyers were unconvinced. 'Covert surveillance' was called for. The recording, coming in and out of her house, the visits to the supermarkets and the hospital appointment, gave utterly conflicting evidence.

Here she is on Tuesday, struggling around Tesco's with a basket in her left hand carrying all the shopping bags back home with her left hand, and struggling with her left hand to turn the key of the front door. Two days later, here she is going round Budgen's with a basket full of groceries in her right hand, the hand that is meant to be so painful, she has no difficulty lugging home bags of shopping shared equally between each hand and turning the key of the front door with her right hand.

This didn't make sense. Was she telling the truth? It all became clear when she came to view the video and walked in with her identical twin who was also her housemate.

The case settled out of court.

> For what avails
> Valour or strength, though matchless, quell'd with pain
> Which all subdues, and makes remiss the hands
> Of Mightiest. Sense of pleasure we may well
> Spare out of life perhaps, and not repine,
> But live content, which is the calmest life:
> But pain is perfect misery, the worst
> Of evils, and excessive, overturns
> All patience.

John Milton. Paradise Lost. Book VI 456/464

Clinical pictures of basic signs

We presented a variety of other symptoms and signs in our 'taxonomical classification'. We now demonstrate some of these with a few more clinical pictures taken from RSD UK members. Let us start with a swollen left foot.

Swelling. There are two types of swelling, one you can see and one you cannot; both are real. We refer to the second as a 'phantom perception', but this is not imagined. It is not a ghost, an apparition, a spirit or a spectre and the patient is rational, sensible and sane. Examples of real and phantom swelling can be seen in Figs 9, 10, pg iv.

Trophic changes. Let us now examine trophic changes where the limb starts to claw. Feet turn in towards the middle and bend at the wrist. Hands may do the same and claw or hook. Hands and feet may shake uncontrollably.

For examples of trophic changes see Figs 9, 10 & 11 [pgs iv, v] where you can see the signs are very variable. They are variable with time, for an individual, and they vary between sufferers. This is not unusual in medicine. Appendicitis can be silent without symptoms or signs and at the other extreme the appendix may have perforated into the bowel and you are close to death. It does make life harder for all.

It helps to have a 'test', an absolute means of checking the diagnosis and sorting it from others that may appear similar, comparable or related. Before we get to what may cause CRPS and how to test for it in a laboratory here are some rashes that may accompany the disease.

Strange rashes are an overlooked feature of CRPS and some examples are shown in Figs 12 –18, pgs vi – ix..

A variety of skin problems are associated with CRPS. Here is a description of one person's experience. We believe it to be common, but the medical literature is sparse.

"When the pain in the arm gets to a certain 'pitch' I start itching – it follows a regular pattern despite what started the increased pain.

35

I start itching on the left wrist, then fingers – I can't scratch it and it often brings tears of frustration as it is so painful; I can though sort of press down on it with my other hand to try to stop the sensations. Itching then starts on my other arm on the wrist then the fingers. Around the same time the part of my neck that was the main site of the original pain (following cervical surgery) itches badly, this starts to get inflamed and the itching turns to an intense itching pain. The feet start next – it is horrible as they are sort of numb and not mine anyway – the itching starts on the ankles, they get very swollen and I have to scratch them. The last area to start itching badly is the bottom of my spine – this also gets very inflamed and I scratch furiously often making the bottom of my back bleed – no matter how hard I try not to scratch I can't stop and often I have been in tears because I need to scratch my better hand, the feet, my neck and back but I cant get to all of them at once."

"After the itching subsides (normally in a day or so) the pain is more intense for a few days with swelling on the bad hand/arm and inflammation on my neck, the feet and my back. Have you had others describe intense itching like this? It annoys everyone around me as I don't seem to be able to stop scratching."

"It would be easy for me to say "the rashes always start when I try to use the arm or hand too much, but it's not that clear-cut".

"The pain sometimes has an odd 'bumpy' feeling with 'hotspots'. I can't think of a better way to describe it. Where there are very hot tight bits on the skin and underneath those bits there is a 'wet' feeling and it is when this happens that the rashes happen."

"The rash starts usually near to the wrist and looks like tiny pinprick red spots, these get bigger and other clusters start appearing on the inside of that forearm until it is all red, but not all of it has the blistering rash part of it. The skin gets very hot. The little spots then start to blister and pop. The blistering and popping can be quite rapid taking only minutes but normally it takes a few hours for the rash to start to pop. After the popping the rash stings badly then starts to dry up – then the skin goes even tighter and hotter. A variable time later, days, maybe weeks, the scabs dry and fall off leaving the arm looking red for a few days or weeks before it goes back to normal.

"The rash normally only goes up to just around the elbow. After having a steroid injection in my shoulder joint I got the same rash on my shoulder joint; the doctor wasn't sure whether to put that down to an allergic reaction or an odd RSD reaction.

"The time the GP watched the blisters form and pop was around four years ago. It was the first time it had covered the entire forearm, before it had just been on my fingers and wrist. On day one he drew a line in pen on that arm to show where the rash extended to. On day two the line was approx two centimetres further all the way around and on day three I got sent to the dermatology clinic. Enough; I was accused of causing them myself."

This is sadly very common. All the rashes shown have been considered at some time by a health professional to be self inflicted or infected.

Spontaneous sub orbital haemorrhage with oedema in a young woman with predominant upper limb CRPS. It started on the involved side and after two days was present on the other

"The rash never itches until it starts healing - it burns badly and the pain is a hotter intense pain on top of the normal pain. It itches a bit after it has gone dry after the blisters have popped." See Figs 14,15 & 17, pgs vii & viii.

"The hairs on my arm originally went very long and black, then I had about two years with no hairs at all on that arm; now they are – just had a look – not as many as my other arm, longer but not darker or standing up."

We know of one medical report on rashes in the dermatology scientific literature looking at eight patients. All had oedema as a cause of swelling. Two had a blistering eruption; these are called bullae, the pleural of bulla. Two had a purpura- like dermatitis which stained the skin.

The word purpura means bleeding into the skin and you can't 'blanche' (lighten) it by pressing down with a glass slide: That's the test. Dermatitis means inflammation in the skin. When a biopsy was taken from a patient with a 'bulla' it did not suggest an influx of immune cells, which is important if you want to know why it happens.

We see these rashes quite frequently and others beside. One common one seems to be very small tense blisters called vesicles often on the sides of fingers that itch. They come and go. Please let us know of any rashes you may get and pictures so we can improve this book. If you have had a biopsy, which we would not necessarily recommend in case the trauma flares, you let us know the result. Thanks. Here are some severe rashes. See Figs 14 – 17 pgs vii, viii.

So what triggers CRPS?

A few patients seem to have an insult so small they have forgotten, but most tell us of a clear injury or medical problem. See Fig 19, pg ix.

Common traumas include:

Chemical burns, electrical injuries.

Bullet and sharp object injuries (occasionally blood sampling).

Blunt or lacerating injuries. Vibration injury. Heavy drilling. Neck injury.

Infection involving nerves (shingles).

Other medical conditions that affect nerves, or blood vessels all of which have nerves, include:

Multiple Sclerosis. Diabetes with nerve damage (diabetic neuropathy). Coronary artery insufficiency and heart attacks.

Surgery particularly involving:

Neck, Hand, wrist, knee, foot, ankle, bowel, bladder and sex organs.

And lots more

Making a diagnosis: laboratory tests

The best way to make a firm diagnosis in medicine is to have available a test that is both 'sensitive' and 'specific'. CRPS does not have one and that hampers and slows down a diagnosis. It all comes down to clinical experience. You match the symptoms with the signs and compare them to all the variable characteristics of the syndrome as understood at present. You use tests to rule out other diagnoses and to get some support for your opinion.

Let us expand on the meaning of sensitive and specific. Here is an example from rheumatology practice, gout. You will see in a moment why we choose gout as an example.

People with acute gout have a few days of agonising pain. They cannot put the foot to the ground if the big toe is involved. Bedclothes are agony. They are fearful, irritable and easily angered. They feel unwell and may have a temperature. The foot is red and hot, and sometimes the whole foot is swollen.

Does this sound a bit like CRPS? Yes, and it is a common misdiagnosis in CRPS of the foot in the early and acute stages. The poorly feeling, the temperature, the swelling, might suggest an infection.

Quite a few diseases look similar. The doctor faced with this diagnostic difficulty may play safe and prescribe an antibiotic as an infection is a diagnosis that could cause the most immediate trouble. He would then tell you to rest it and return if it gets no better.

He does however have a test or two that can help with the diagnosis; these are laboratory-based. He can take a blood sample to measure uric acid. Uric acid levels are closely linked to the disease. They are raised in classical gout so the test is often helpful. However it may be normal during an acute attack, and not high in chronic disease.

It may be raised in someone without disease. The test therefore has limited **specificity**, as it can't pick out disease from non-disease. It has limited **sensitivity** because it does not select all sufferers. It is a good test for some but misleading for others. See Fig 21, 22 pg x.

What laboratory tests we have for CRPS have even less specificity and sensitivity so none are diagnostic. This is what we have at present. See images showing gout and infection, both looking like CRPS Figs 23, 24.

Thermographs.

"The only reason I had this done was because I took part in some research at a hospital and part of the research was looking at temperature within the affected area. The first thermal image I had done, I remember feeling quite shocked by it because the temperature that it showed was very low in my arm.

This was quite confusing because I thought my arm was burning. It made quite an impact on me and also my GP as obviously he had this image in front of him; a blue arm. When he looked at mine it was more often red than blue."

"The thermograph made it real for other people. People that hadn't seen the swelling or the shiny red blistering skin could now see something. That certainly helped to show the people that it's not just a pain condition. There's something tangible there that they could relate to. A thermograph is so simple. It's in colour as well. So if it's in colour it's got to be true. Anything in black and white is lies!" "He took pictures of my left arm which was good, and then pictures of my right arm and also pictures of them together to see if there was a difference in temperature between the two arms."

"The test is painless, though the room is air-conditioned and cold, and it takes about forty five minutes. Most of this time spent is stabilising your temperature in the room."

A thermograph is a sensitive test.   Most patients have differences between the arms or legs and these are much greater than normal differences. It is not a specific test; other diseases can cause differences, but to be fair these can be easily picked up by either a full clinical history or examination or other tests that are not positive in CRPS.

All in all, and when linked to the clinical exam, the test is useful and we use it clinically to aid diagnosis, to assess progress, and for research. Figs 22, 23, pg xi.

X Rays

Since Professor W. Röntgen's discovery that X-rays (December 28, 1895) can identify bony structures, X-rays have been refined for their use in medical imaging. X-rays are especially helpful in the detection of pathology of the skeletal system, but are also valuable for detecting some disease processes in soft tissue.

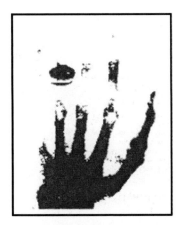 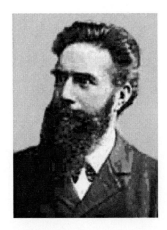

First X-ray image by W Roentgen.

We use x-rays for more than one reason, but primarily to exclude other pathologies. These include a fracture, or a bone infection. In CRPS we look for a rather strange pattern of local bone thinning that may come and go and this is reasonably, but not completely, specific. This 'regional osteoporosis' may be caused by other conditions; the 'commonest is an acute nerve death in diabetes. This can look just like CRPS and in some ways it is the same disease, though not classified as such.

An X-ray is not a sensitive test as many patients don't have osteoporosis, or don't have it at the time they are X-rayed.

"With the X-rays they couldn't find anything major wrong except the muscle and soft tissue damage caused by the injury."

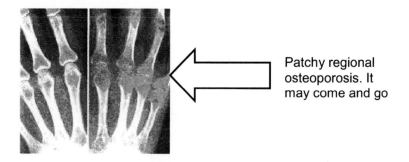

Patchy regional osteoporosis. It may come and go

A Bone Scan

The test is performed to identify abnormal processes involving the bone. Some, but not all patients show enhanced activity in the affected part. The test is only sensitive in the first six months, and then only picks up half of the cases.

A radiotracer, a 'radionuclide', which is very weakly radioactive, is injected through a vein. As it decays, gamma radiation is emitted, which is detected by a camera that scans your body. The camera detects how much radiotracer collects in the bones. The procedure can take a little while, but will not cause you difficulties

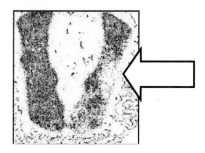

A bone scan in CRPS of the left foot, the foot on your right in this book.

Ultrasound

Ultrasound imaging, also called ultrasound scanning or sonography, is a method of obtaining images from the muscles and tendons using high-frequency sound waves. The reflected sound wave echoes are recorded as a real-time visual image. Because ultrasound images are captured in this way they can show movement. No x-ray is involved in ultrasound imaging.

We use ultrasound to see if ligaments and muscles are torn. The test requires an expert both in the procedure and the analysis

"The test was quick, easy and safe. I could see my torn ligament, it wasn't badly enough torn for the pain I had, so they said this tear could well be complicated by CRPS and they would get me physiotherapy fast. I did it for ages every day and at home and all is fine now. It was scary though because up to then I was getting worse all the time. My orthopaedic surgeon was great."

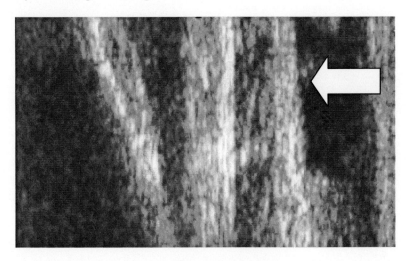

A tear in the Achilles tendon.

Electromyogram and Nerve Conduction Studies.

The term 'electro diagnostic testing' covers a whole spectrum of specialized tests, including the Electromyogram (EMG), and nerve conduction studies (NCS). Many rheumatological problems involving nerves or muscles require these tests to exclude other pathologies or establish, in type 2 CRPS, the extent of nerve damage.

The test system uses many 'machines that go ping' including a computer, monitor, amplifier, loudspeaker, and stimulator to see and hear how muscles and nerves are working. In the EMG examination a small needle is inserted into muscles, both where you are having symptoms and further away.Muscle tissue is normally electrically silent at rest but when the muscle is voluntarily contracted, (electrical signals) begin to appear. Patterns of action potentials are altered in diseases of muscle and nerves and may be abnormal in CRPS

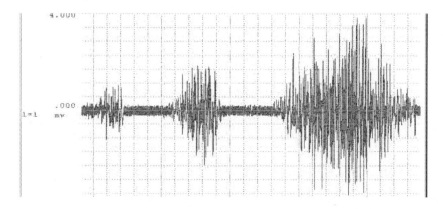

Electrical discharges in muscle

Nerve conduction studies are undertaken to monitor the functioning nerves and muscles in your body. The examiner places electrodes on your skin over the muscles being tested. Using a stimulator to deliver a small electrical current to your skin, and near to your nerves, causes them to fire. The electrical signals produced by nerves and muscles are then analysed.

Both motor nerves which activate muscles and sensory nerves that can generate pain are tested. The small nerve fibres that are likely to be responsible for many of the signs we have discussed cannot be tested.

NCS can evaluate the severity of medium or large nerve damage. A focal neuropathy is when a single nerve is damaged somewhere at a site along its course.

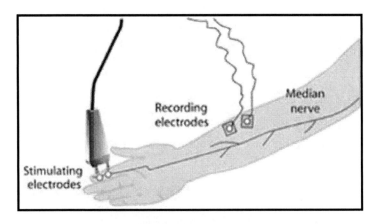

Nerve Conduction Studies

"I had nerve conduction studies. If any one tells you they don't hurt, they lie; they do."

They will hurt more in CRPS with allodynic symptoms, for reasons we have discussed and will discuss again... as one of the authors, Catherine, has just discovered. Here she is again exaggerating it all!
"The test was brutal: sadists."

The test is occasionally used later in the disease process to rule out nerve entrapment complications caused by trophic changes and oedema. More often these can be diagnosed by a specialist in the clinic.

Measurements of sweating

A variety of techniques are available to accurately measure the increased sweating (sudomotor dysfunction), which may be more on the affected than on the normal side. It can be fairly easily witnessed clinically perhaps with warm stimulation and is rarely measured by quantitative techniques apart from as research tests. It is sensitive but not very specific, but in the correct clinical context and having excluded mimics of CRPS, it may be useful.

A lie detector test or polygraph works on the same principle and measures sweat output as one measure of autonomic activity (sympathetic) which changes when we lie. If a person is lying, his heart rate, blood pressure, respiratory rate and electro-dermal activity (sweatiness) increases and enough to be measured.

Measuring Blood Flow

This is measured by a technique such as plethysmography or laser flowmetry. Blood flow is altered in CRPS and differently in acute and chronic CRPS. Investigators suggest this is due to alterations in brain autonomic activity; changes seem to occur almost minute by minute.

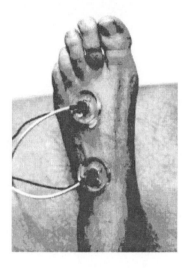

Laser Doppler flowmetry

Dexa Scan (Dexa) or Dual X- Ray Absorptiometry

This test is not used to make a diagnosis in CRPS, but is helpful to asses a possible complication after immobility, 'osteoporosis' or thin bones. A Dexa scan is the newest and the most precise technique for evaluating osteoporosis which can be local in CRPS or more general if immobility stops movement or weight bearing.

A Dexa test measures the density (or thickness) of your bones. It does this by sending a thin beam of x-rays through bones. The amount of radiation is very small. Based on how much the x-rays change after passing through your bones, a picture of your skeleton will be generated and an osteoporosis score calculated. No anaesthesia is required as this procedure is painless. You lie, clothed, on a cushioned table. The arm of the DEXA machine passes over your body taking the measurements over ten minutes. The test is interpreted for you by the specialist after comparing with reference standards. See Fig 27 pg xii

The lower your bone density, the higher your risk of bone fractures. General exercise and weight bearing are important in maintaining bone strength. Being a woman, having an early menopause, a family history of osteoporosis, a poor diet, smoking, alcohol excess and other serious illnesses are other risk factors. The disease can be treated or controlled by drugs quite safely.

The concept of central pain

You will have heard the expression 'it's all in the mind'. Perhaps someone has suggested that your CRPS pain is! If you are a carer maybe you have considered the possibility too. It's clear that sometimes health professionals suggest it either directly or indirectly.

The expression is harmful to the sufferer as it has negative connotations. If, by the mind however, you mean the brain or central nervous system, then you are probably correct.

The brain itself does not feel pain, but it can generate pain elsewhere if injured. A variety of medical names are given to these phenomena depending on where the injury occurred. [In this context it is also known as the Thalamic Pain Syndrome, Dejerine-Roussy Syndrome, Posterior Thalamic Syndrome, Retrolenticular Syndrome and Central Post-Stroke Syndrome.]

The Central Pain Syndrome Alliance (CPSA) website says "It can be a steady, sometimes deep burning, aching, cutting, tearing sensation. Central Pain Syndrome may be mixed with sudden, excruciating shots of pain. It is often mixed with other distracting sensations like cold giving tingling, a 'pins and needles' effect, a ballooning sensation, a throbbing feeling, and the reaction of a dental probe on a raw nerve."

Is this not nearly exactly the same as our descriptions? Yes it is identical. Nerve injury or neuropathic states can also cause a central pain syndrome and we believe that CRPS is another disease that falls under this broad heading.

This is what they say triggers Central Pain Syndrome.
"We have defined the following things that we can call 'triggers' to start or increase one's sensations and pain levels: Movement, daily activity, exposure to sun, cold, breezes, air conditioning, barometer changes, weather (both hot and cold), rain, snow.

Others include real pain or swelling, stress, anger, depression, touches of another person, blanket, clothes, splints; tiredness, sudden movement (for example yawning) and other involuntary movements like sneezing, being startled, fear, vibration, even riding in a car."

These are again the same triggers members of RSD UK tell us set off their CRPS.

So the answer is yes, it is all in the 'mind' and only an ignorant Aussie would call you a 'whinging pom'. Now we will explore how this comes about.

The Nervous System both peripheral and central

The story starts with a Frenchman, René Descartes, who is often called the 'father' of modern philosophy. Many who study pain science would consider him our founder too

He was a philosopher and an academic who drew a distinction between the mind and the body. This is now called 'Cartesian dualism'. He suggested that the mind and body were two entirely separate things though scientists now believe that no such distinction exists.

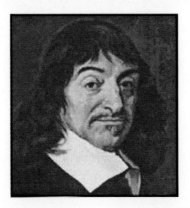

René Descartes (French 1596-1650)

René Descartes identified the pain pathway from the periphery (the foot) to the spinal cord and the brain. Until then pain was thought to be felt in your heart.

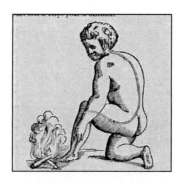

René Descartes has drawn a central and peripheral nervous pathway, but he never saw nerves and they had not been described. Quite remarkable.

In medicine we subdivide the nervous system into the peripheral nervous system and the central nervous system or CNS.

The CNS includes the brain and the spinal cord extending from lower in your back to the base of the brain at the bottom of the skull. There are millions of fine nerves almost everywhere in your body and at the end of these are receptors. A receptor is similar to a socket and responds to a specific input from the area around. There are visceral receptors from internal organs and somatosensory receptors for the rest of you, muscles ligaments and so on. This is what they look like in a diagram for medical students.

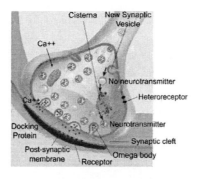

Complicated eh?!
From www.colorado.edu

50

The major input systems are our five senses: touch/pain, vision, taste, smell, and hearing. Sensory receptors are classified according to the type of energy they can detect and respond to. Here they are. Please think about them as possible entry points for stimulating allodynic pain in CRPS, itself an example of a central pain syndrome.

Peripheral receptors

The Somatosensory receptors detecting stimuli in your limbs include:

Mechanoreceptors and Thermoreceptors.

Nociceptors (derived from Latin-nocēre, to hurt) which respond to damage and send the signals to the CNS where they may be turned into a pain like perceptions

Proprioceptors (derived from Latin proprius, meaning 'one's own' and 'perception') telling us where we are and sending to the information to the CNS where it is usually stored usually subconsciously

Mechanoreceptors (mechanical receptors) for hearing balance and stretching

Photoreceptors (photons or light) for light

Chemoreceptors (chemical) for smell and taste, as well as internal sensors in the digestive and circulatory/vascular systems

Thermoreceptors (Thermo is heat) for changes in temperature

Electroreceptors (Electrical) to detect electrical currents in the surrounding environment

All the nerves outside your central nervous system create the peripheral nervous system. Its job is to spread information from your brain and spinal cord to the rest of your body and back again.

It is divided into three parts. The **motor system** controls movement following signals *from* the CNS. The **sensory system** transmits sensations *to* the CNS. It also transmits information from your joints, ligaments and muscles as to where you are, and where your joints are (proprioception). Much of this information is stored in your brain at a sub conscious level.

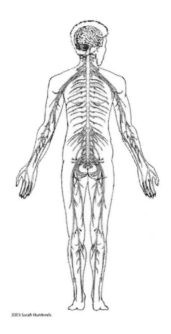

The brain, spinal cord and peripheral nerves (a few) coming from it and going everywhere. The brain and spinal cord make up the Central Nervous System or CNS.

Artist Sarah Huntrods From roadhunter@nucleus.com

The third peripheral system is the **autonomic nervous system** which is mostly outside of our control. This system is subdivided into the **sympathetic system** and **parasympathetic system**. These two automatic units also send signals to the brain and the brain sends signals back down the spinal cord. We discuss where in the brain later.

The sympathetic system is involved in 'flight and fright' or 'stressing out' responses.

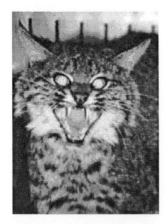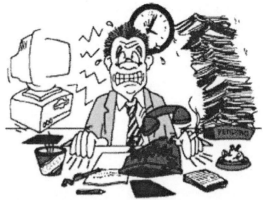

Frightened and about to flee or perhaps attack.
Image from www.chintiminiwildlife.org and www.ninaspencer.com

With acute sympathetic activity senses are keener, your memory is sharper, and you are less sensitive to pain. With chronic stimulation, as above, this advantage is lost, indeed reversed. The text box describes what the sympathetic autonomic system does and we explain the brain centres involved in more detail later.

During the **'flight or fright'** response in man and wild animals, the brain engages in considerable activity. The *amygdala* signals the *hypothalamus*, which then drives the sympathetic nervous system. The peripheral autonomic nerves release the body, either adrenalin (epinephrine if from USA) or noradrenalin (norepinephrine) which stimulates many organs to prepare for flight.

The adrenal gland is also stimulated to release compounds including cortisol, a steroid into the blood for a prolonged stimulatory effect. The heart rate increases. Glucose, a sugar, is released from the liver for energy. Bronchi dilate opening the lungs and the pupils dilate. When a **'fight or fright'** response doesn't work, animals becomes very frustrated or distressed, it may adopt the 'conservation-withdrawal' response. An animal in conservation-withdrawal will appear quiet and depressed.

If levels of cortisol rise to a certain level, several areas of the brain, principally the *hippocampus,* tell the *hypothalamus* to turn off cortisol production. This is the proper feedback response. One function of the hippocampus is memory formation and storage Excessive cortisol, too high for too long can make it difficult to think or retrieve long-term memories.

That's why people get confused in a crisis. Too much cortisol prevents the brain from laying down a new memory, or from accessing already existing memories.

This also explains why overstressed adults taking their annual holidays with the kids behave like complete 'plonkers' in airports and hotels.

Who says science is not relevant?

The parasympathetic system plays its part in 'rest and digest' reactions.

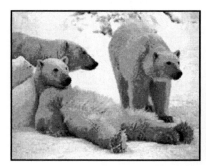 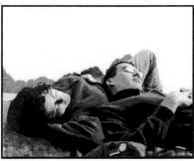

'Rest and digest' or 'chilling out' is the parasympathetic systems business.

From web.syr.edu. And www.semisable.com.

Your parasympathetic nervous system does more or less the opposite of the sympathetic system.

Complimentary physicians would say it maintains our Yin and Yang type balance. If the sympathetic is Yin then the parasympathetic is Yang.

Yang restores your energy. It directs blood to your digestive tract helping you to digest food. It maintains your blood pressure, heart rate and breathing rate at a low level. The intestines expand and the gut and intestines activate. The parasympathetic system assists in removing metabolic waste products such as adrenaline and lactic acid. Its actions are generated by the chemical neurotransmitter, acetylcholine.

In CRPS the altered blood vessel responses are attributed to autonomic dysfunction. The excessive sweating indicates an amplified skin sympathetic response, which you can measure by the sweating tests we described. The deep heat feeling and burning pain is, we think, coming from a cross wiring in the spinal cord, between the sympathetic nervous system and the peripheral nerves system. Blood vessels can feel pain and heat which explains why the 'pain feeling' is often a deep pain.

More on the Central Nervous System

The Brain—is wider than the Sky—
for—put them side by side—
the one the other will contain
with ease—and you—beside—

Emily Dickinson 1830-1886.

Your ears, eyes and nose also transmit information about where you are. They can detect potentially dangerous threats and transmit the information directly to the brain. The brain analyses much of the information in the lower brain section, which is in an evolutionary sense, older and more concerned with reflex and autonomic behaviour critical for survival in the broadest sense.

It is divided into two, the brain stem at the bottom and above it the midbrain. It transmits the information gathered to the upper newer brain 'the cerebrum' which again subdivides into parts. Many pain pathways are networked between the lower and upper brain areas. Not all areas of the brain are involved, but many are. This is what is meant by a network, a set of connections between different anatomical areas that can also communicate with other networks.

A network is merely a system that connects various elements; it can be simple or complex. The degree of complexity is dependent on the number of basic contributors and the number of assets that they will share with the system. Consider a family network. One mother, one father and two teenagers being a standard network that shifts rapidly from stability to chaos. They live in an interconnected fashion and of course communicate with other networks, some more crucial than others; neighbours, work, leisure and so on. The basic family network can be influenced by slight disturbances in another linked network. The father's boss dies, he is promoted and the family is now changed, perhaps a little, perhaps permanently, perhaps for the better, perhaps not. The daughter becomes pregnant and instability may ensue or not.

Here are some network designs. The question is what basic design does acute pain belong to? Is chronic pain an extension of this network or a different beast all together? What has happened to transform a usually stable network into an unstable or chaotic one as appears to be the case in CRPS?

By studying 'theoretical network topologies' or maps we hope to construct ideas that allow us to test for the dominant influences and points or nodes where change may be most effective.

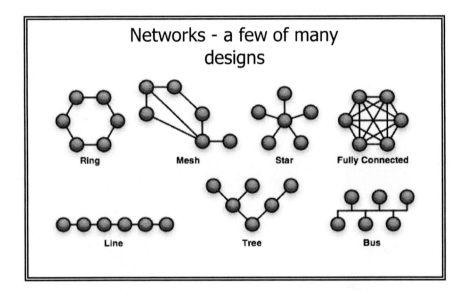

As we discuss the brain in a little more detail try to consider the various anatomical structures as the green balls or nodes. Science originally tried to explain their functions as line networks. Organ one talks to two and so on. It is much more complex than that as anybody with a family understands. Some systems work as stars, others as trees or rings. "Trees" may be joined to a "mesh" and then to "trees" and the final pathway out may be a "bus" or a "star". The potential for small hiccups having large and unexpected effects can be worsened by complex networks, but similarly the effect can be reduced if there are spare or back-up systems. The human brain consists of around 10^{11} (100,000,000,000) neurons which are highly interconnected with around 10^{14} (1,000,000,000,000,000) connections. We are talking 'complex' as the number of combinations is near infinite, making us not as daft as we seem. Figs 25, 26 pg vii

The sensory nervous system transmits information about any potentially painful insult up the spinal cord. It is processed in the brain stem and integrated with other evolutionary old systems. It is transmitted further up to the midbrain and then, after further processing, on to the cerebrum and the cerebellum. Information is then sent all around the network and back down to create the responses and perceptions. All is very complicated, but it gets worse. Figs 30, 31

Man has a large cerebrum, dogs smaller, reptiles miniscule; all these species feel pain in some form or another, but not necessarily as we do. Rats squeal easily enough if hurt, so do Spring Peeper frogs who throw their voices to distract the predator.

We would not want to be lobsters heading for boiling water either, though it is unlikely they would feel pain precisely as we would. However, there is no reason for thinking they don't feel it as unpleasant distress. UK chef Gordon Ramsey explains exactly how to kill live lobsters and how it makes him feel.

> "You always feel better after killing something. I do... stab the head of a lobster. You feel all the better for it... God knows how many I've killed... plunge them into boiling court bouillon, and their tails flip up and they scream and you can hear their claws scraping on the sides, and I got great pleasure out of that."
> (The Independent Magazine UK, 12/10/2003).

Here is a quote from a child with CRPS

.

> *"It feels like someone poured petrol on my leg and set it on fire"*

More on pain in the mind

Now we mean a CNS network

"The very problem of mind and body suggests division; I do not know of anything so disastrously affected by the habit of division as this particular theme. In its discussion are reflected the splitting off from each other of religion, morals and science; the divorce of philosophy from science and of both from the arts of conduct. The evils which we suffer in education, in religion, in the materialism of business and the aloofness of "intellectuals" from life, in the whole separation of knowledge and practice -- all testify to the necessity of seeing mind-body as an integral whole."

John Dewey: 1859 - 1952

What is your mind? You know what we propose but here are some definitions from the Web.

"The human consciousness that originates in the brain and is manifested especially in thought, perception, emotion, will, memory, and imagination."

"The collective conscious and unconscious processes, in a sentient organism that direct and influence mental and physical behaviour."

Some consider it to be the same as your soul. This is quite a different entity as defined this way.

"The spiritual nature of humans, regarded as immortal, separable from the body at death, and susceptible to happiness or misery in a future state: the disembodied spirit of a dead human."

The mind may produce pain, but scientists know nothing of the soul. So far we have established that pain is produced from sensations that are derived from inputs from the periphery, and processed in the Central Nervous System. The CNS creates perceptions that are expressed in consciousness. It does this via interlinking networks of variable complexity.

Pain that you can anticipate is a slightly different process from sensory pain signals you cannot, as networks can be recruited in anticipation. Pains from pinches that you might make to your own skin are processed somewhat differently from those of strangers and particularly from those when you are taken unaware. This is an example of one insult, giving rise to at least three different perceptions and a larger number of dissimilar behaviours.

Stimuli go up from the periphery and come down as the perception of pain reasonably anatomically close to where the sensory insult commenced. But could pain perceptions come direct to the brain from other sensory inputs that connect directly to the brain? The eyes, ears and nose we have mentioned. In other words could I startle you and give you a pain in a localisable anatomical site?

This is such an important point that we say it twice. Could pain perceptions come direct to the brain from other sensory inputs that connect directly to the brain? If the brain was all wound up from an ongoing event in the periphery, could visual or auditory stimuli feed into and stimulate the network and generate the perception of pain. To go another step, could the mere threat of being touched or the thought of moving cause pain?

Well, you would have to be mad to consider it. Pain would surely be in your mind. Not so, we hear it all the time. We have been largely ignoring this symptom and the accompanying signs for years or responding negatively. We have read some descriptions of odd responses already… and we call it 'pain behaviour'.

Pain behaviour

Considered, by some, an abnormal psychological reaction to pain but considered by us to be a near invariable response to allodynia. Doctors assess it in the clinic and may try to observe you at other times. They study you under the five categories of 'guarding, touching, sounds, words, and facial expression.' If we see discrepancies of behaviour in different settings, or responses that are inappropriate to the stimulus, we may send patients to psychologists and psychiatrists presuming they are somehow 'round the bend'. We call it aberrant pain behaviour.

It is however a fact that allodynic pain is always associated with observable pain behaviours; it is the nature of the beast. Psychologists and others if knowledgeable about pain help, not by confirming madness, but by explaining the process. They then assist by reconditioning the system in tandem with other health professionals. Here is an example of what might be called disproportionate pain behaviour, though it is not...

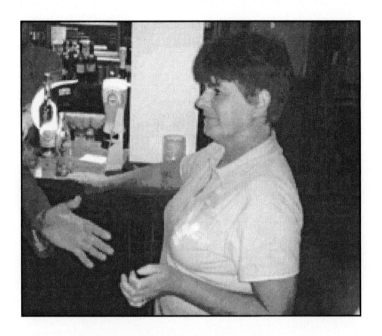

An author conducting an experiment in the bar.

Catherine is showing 'pain behaviour'.

Here we show allodynia in an extreme form. David (author), in a bar, is examining Catherine's hand (authoress). It seems a normal enough colour at this moment, but it feels cold. He is bringing his left hand to as close to Catherine's CRPS left hand as she can accept.

Look at her face and her posture. At this point Catherine is starting to guard and not only feels apprehensive, but experiences more pain in the hand. Her best friend could touch the hand, just. Catherine could touch her own. Each feeling of pain was different. The hand is clawed, but this is not permanent and varies with stimuli.

More pain dialogues and stories

Before we move to dialogues and stories that illustrate much of this let us sidestep and tell you from where we borrowed the idea of dialogues. It was Dava Sobel, authoress, scientific correspondent and patron of the charity BIRD attached to our institute, who indirectly promoted the idea of this book explaining arguments through dialogues and narratives.

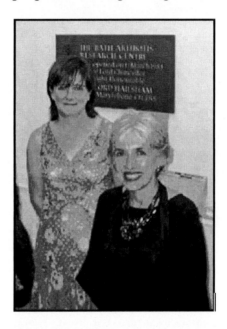

Ms. Dava Sobel with Ms. Rachel Edwards (left) of "Rachel's story"

In her book 'Galileo's Daughter' we hear plenty about her father Galileo Galilei who had problems with the Church following his adaptation of the telescope. His pointed it at the heavens and concluded the earth was not the central point in the solar system; it was the sun.

To put over this idea, which put him in conflict with religious creed, he used three fictitious characters. Two strongly expressed the opposite view and one, presented as less than clever, argued Galileo's true position. He lost the argument, but all who read the book presumed Galileo was the 'not so clever' one and many agreed with his argument. The Inquisition was displeased with Galileo's deception.

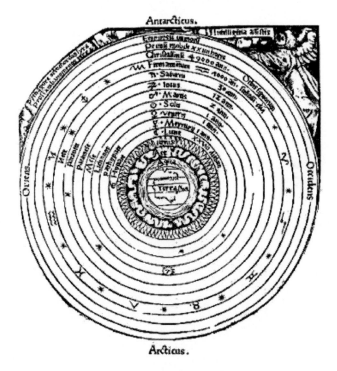

From Aristotle *Libri de caelo* (1519).
From Duke University Library USA.

So where is the central point, the sun, in CRPS and what is orbiting what?

Dissecting 'allodynic pain states' carefully is no academic whim. It is important as the analysis may provide clues, which allow for a theory to be proposed and then tested. This may then help in designing new treatments, either pharmacologically-based, or not.
Here are four dialogues from memory, they relate to the language of pain and we will use language as our starting point as they may indicate nodes in the network which may allow us to find the central point:

"Sarah, please do the washing up for once," I beg.
"Dad, you're a pain in the neck", she mutters, sloping off.

This is no mystical pain which has been transmitted by sorcery, but a figure of speech. Not all societies would use such an expression. Racial groups, different religious faiths, and children in particular describe pain very differently. A few, translating from their own language, will say that a very severe pain is pain everywhere. They actually mean it's an overwhelming pain and this can cause confusion for medical staff.

A young daughter, during 'the dreadful threes' sobs to her Mum "Mum I have tummy ache". Mum's a GP and little Caroline has an ear infection, 'otitis media.'

Is this a poor representation of Caroline's sense of internal space, known as her egocentric representation? Is it adrift due to an immature brain? Or is it just simple, poorly developed language? Well, it's an odd language error and an unlikely explanation, as so many similarly aged children say precisely the same.

Now, for a fictitious conversation that takes place between a young adult, Jonathan, and his friend Richard. Richard is unemployed. A few weeks back as a car passenger he is involved in a shunting accident. His head goes forward, his neck back, but there is no head rest. He is shaken, but not stirred.

"Whiplash probably", says his doctor. "It would be best to check an x-ray... all fine", he announces.

Richard is not so sure; he has had a slowly expanding gnawing ache in his arm.

"The pain is difficult to describe", he tells Jonathan. "And now I ache all over, maybe I roughed up more than I thought."

He sees an advert for claiming liability damages. He reads it to Jonathan. "You have sustained an injury in an accident that was not your fault and would like to make a claim for personal injury... Symptoms might include pain in the neck area and a stiff sore neck, pain in the muscles in the shoulders. Headaches and migraines may occur. You may have numbness or 'pins and needles' in the shoulders, arms and hands... you may ache more generally."

Richard starts to experience these.

Doctors are uncertain about whiplash injuries. In countries with stricter compensation rules the frequency of reporting this diagnosis drops. On the other hand, spinal trauma, as in brain trauma, can directly cause pain to be perceived as we have seen in the 'Central Pain Syndrome'.

Could the concern about Richard's financial situation and his lack of work contribute to his growing preoccupation with his pain? A pain attended to expands, and distraction suppresses pain. Indeed, major tissue trauma on a battlefield may not be immediately associated with pain despite all the sensory signals the nerves are sending to the brain.

Many consider that CRPS pains are similar to whiplash injuries, namely overplayed and occasionally fabricated and then they look at the patients' pain behaviours to substantiate this view.

None of these dialogues are the same however as these from CRPS sufferers.

"The pain was just so intense, you couldn't touch it and people said 'Well you could wear a glove couldn't you?' but you couldn't put a glove on."

"I am very reluctant for other people like physiotherapists to touch it either so we're all in a 'Catch 22' aren't we?"

"I did touch it, yeah. And that, again that was so confusing because when I touched it, it felt in one way like you touch your lip after an anaesthetic at the dentist and it gave an electric shock feeling, like a great big jolt."

"I went down to see this doctor and he prodded and poked and I mean by then my leg was unbearable, every touch was like I wanted to go through the roof..."

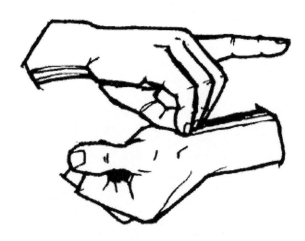

Pinching and prodding.
Do to others as you would be done by - don't do it.

"If you touched it with you know just anything soft it feels sharp."
So there you have it. These are not figures of speech; anatomical location is not confused and there is no fabrication or expansion. It is all too similar. These are concise descriptions of allodynia or severe hyperaesthesia. They are created sometimes to mere threats of injury, and then cause a sense of dread.

All these dialogues suggest that the brain is now in the driving seat and generating the pain in response to the smallest of stimuli, many non-noxious. You will again be struck more by the remarkable similarities of these dialogues than the differences. You will also notice the emotional aspects to the pain perception and how disproportionate this is to the signal that created it. It is the job of qualitative scientists to collect and catalogue these. The quantitative scientists then decode these into potential brain areas and constructs testing systems.

More words - pain and emotion

Over the last few years we have been patiently collecting the words people use to describe there symptoms and we described some earlier. This has been done by others, but perhaps not comprehensively in CRPS. One of the first to collect pain words to assist in understanding the mechanism of pain was Professor R Melzack at McGill University

Montreal, Quebec, Canada. He devised a questionnaire consisting of seventy eight descriptive words suggested by patients with different pain states. The words are divided into three subsets.

Sensory, affective and evaluative words. Some words describe the **sensory** component, others the **affective** and the third, the **evaluative.**

Sensory words would be those like throbbing, burning or aching. Others that are different from each other are flickering, jumping, pricking, and sharp, pinching, tugging, hot, tingling, or dull.

Affective words, meaning how they affect you would be tiring, sickening, killing, wretched, unbearable, torturing or blinding.

Evaluative words, that also have affective qualities to a degree, are spreading, penetrating, and piercing.

Patients with CRPS pain score highly for each separate subset, sensory, affective and evaluative. In fact all patients with allodynic pain of central origin score highly in all three subsets and the test is helpful to doctors in diagnosing allodynic states. Mind you, listening to the words that are spontaneously expressed is as good.
We have read many of them already and the affective and evaluative components are very clear. It is however clear from the stories earlier that this 'word test' is often not recognised in clinical practice as a means of suspecting allodynic pain.

Here is a shortened (by us) description of CRPS taken from the Web and put up by an American school girl. It is very moving. She presented it as a speech to her school.

Really Stupid Disease

"I want to tell you about the disease 'Really Stupid Disease'
It's hard to believe it can cause so much grief for a person. Horrible, awful, excruciating pain I suffer from every day. Imagine submerging your foot in a vat of boiling oil.

That, my friends, is a manageable day. Lightning shoots up my calf with shooting pain, extreme temperature changes, complete numbness, and tremendous swelling.

Anyone who has ever experienced a stinger knows how uncomfortable they are. Multiply that pain level by one thousand, and you're near the parking lot of the ballpark I'm playing in. It feels like my foot is on fire."

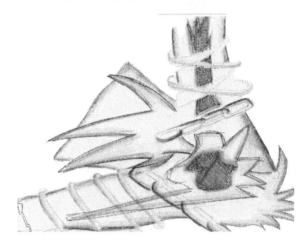

The allodynic pain of CRPS. Stories and pictures help diagnosis

Rejection

And now we illustrate a common problem, that of rejection, to understand the emotional response

"The doctor had no idea what was wrong so she went to an adjoining room to ask the consultant for advice, he saw my notes (the door was open) and said, whilst throwing my notes on to the desk, "With the size of these notes it will be self-inflicted. Discharge her." So I left: My reaction, I cried for days…"

And so would we. Most would not be annoyed with a professional who had no idea as that's common enough in medicine.

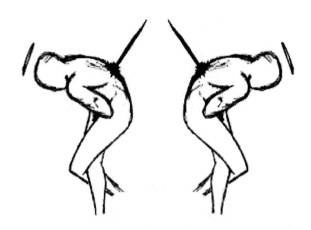

The angels cried tears of blood."
From www.argh.de/archives/

The problem is the cruel dismissal based on ignorance and apathy tinged with spite.

It is harder if you are rejected by your family.

Here is a poem from Heather a member of 'Pain Pals Jr. Kid's Club', a place where children of RSD parents, grandparents, and loved ones can meet others and learn that they are not alone.

THE TERRIBLE, HORRIBLE RSD MONSTER

(An RSD poem by Heather-age 9)

You see her every night
She gives you such a fright.
Don't you dare go near her!
She's NOT very nice.
She'll gobble you up
When she is screaming and crying.
She is on so many medications
That you never know what will go flying.
When she's in a good mood,

She's nice in some ways.
Our lives have been ruined by her RSD.
So, for a cure PLEASE help me pray!!
Let's stop this monster RSD
And bring back my mommy
The way she
Used to be!!!

www.angelfire.com/me2/ rsdpainpals/kidsclub.html

Concentration

Concentration is difficult in this disease, sometimes impossible. There is too much nervous system discharge going on to deal with this book or anything else.

One of us having written the above paused, took a walk and these were thoughts generated expressed as a 'little bit of a true story.'

"My God I have shocking toothache," I say to Sheila.

"To the dentist," she replies.

"Root abscess. Do you brush your teeth regularly?" says Ms. Molarity.

"Sure, every Christmas; I think the word you want is frequently."
Well she cleans it up, having flicked the filling off the tooth cap with no more than a prod and I'm armed with antibiotics, already partially cured, and back in ten days.

"Very nice," she says in the self-congratulatory way we professionals speak if something looks just reasonable. A further cleanse inside and a nice temporary filling that mysteriously made the cavity in my tooth feel smaller.

Three days later. "God help me, this is pounding." I say loudly to Sheila.

"Bloody dentists." I was that close to getting the pliers and yanking the filling off and plenty of abnormal pain behaviours were to be seen.
And so to the dentist, she white coated with syringe in hand. "I can't bear it, no, yes, quick". The job is done.

70

"Off you go and come back in three weeks; the tooth may have to go."
"Hang on, just a quick detour to the lavatory."

This lip feels very swollen. It feels all puffed up, it's bloated, and it feels all inflamed. Has she bashed it? No the mirror shows me it's all in my mind. I turn away and would you believe it, it's swollen, it's not a little bit swollen, and it's out there. No problems, I have had it before, just the anaesthetic; it will pass, it does, and I dribble a bit.

That was a true-ish story; fiction based on some historical fact. The perceptions and emotions are genuine. We believe we describe a common enough experience in the Western world in adults over forty. In the text you see similar emotional outputs to those described in the CRPS dialogues. There was also 'phantom swelling'.

Nobody medically trained finds it hard to explain my responses. An infection around a nerve root in an area with lots of sensory nerves is painful; very painful. Infection in this area creates a long-lasting throbbing pain. A local anaesthetic to the mandibular nerve leaves all with a perception of a swollen lip. The lip is not truly swollen.

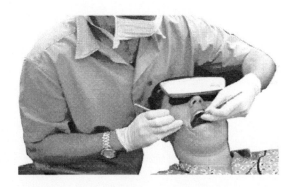

Dental anaesthetic can cause phantom perceptions

So could a patient have a swollen hand, foot or elsewhere, that felt swollen, but wasn't; ... and is it possible that the mechanism was the same, or similar?

Now, those without CRPS should 'take ten' or more and consider how you would feel if you woke one morning with a huge lip, that wasn't, but certainly felt it was. A lip that burnt, throbbed, and gnawed all day.

The feelings come in waves, and are made worse by washing your face. Imagine what it would feel like if all this worsened, if a loved one embraced you, and how you would feel if no-one had ever seen this, and there was no end in sight. Here is the answer.

Anger, frustration, depression, hostility and turning it all around

"Holding on to anger is like grasping a hot coal with the intent of throwing it at someone else; you are the one getting burned."

Buddha

Anger is a harmful emotion. It is very common and it upsets at least two people. It is caused by frustration and maximal when we judge someone else is to blame. Anger is described as 'an emotional, physiological, cognitive internal state'. Importantly it exists separately from the actions it prompts. A chronic state of anger creates hostility. Chronic stimulation of the autonomic system will generate this response.

One common way of expressing anger is to suppress it. This has been called, 'passive-aggressiveness'. It is the act of releasing your anger by being passive. For example you may be tired, unresponsive, tearful, or argumentative. You may be forgetful, clumsy or sick. Another form of concealed anger is 'feeling like a victim' and depression and suicide may follow. We have seen that animals behave similarly here biologists called it the 'conservation-withdrawal' response.

Here is a moving story from the National Pain Foundation that illustrates some of these aspects. It is a part of a story of Cynthia Toussaint who was a ballerina until a trivial injury whilst dancing left her with CRPS.

"Other than my partner John and my mother, no one else stayed in my life. To be fair, I hated the world, everyone and everything. I was watching everyone else move on with their lives," she explains.

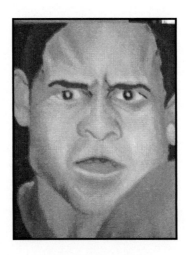

"Anger and Fear"
Artist Christopher Blake; self portrait

"I know that my siblings love me intensely, but they can't handle what's happened to me. Cynthia says that people don't understand how her family could have left and it is easy to explain. There aren't any bad guys here. I understand why they would leave; I think about their anger and their survivor guilt. I think about how different their lives would be if this hadn't happened. They were victims too. The fact that our great family could be destroyed means anyone's can be. Chronic pain really happens to all the family and while some people might come back into your life, you can never be that family again."

Here are other dialogues.

"The pains and everything that you've had; why couldn't it have happened to somebody else? Although it may sound selfish, why me?"

"I've also got a violent temper now which I never had before. I'm having anger management classes now, I never dreamt that I would ever resort to talking to somebody about problems that I had."

"Again I was angry against the system, because I knew there was something wrong with me. I cry loads and I ball and ball and I'll, I'll turn the phones off to be all alone and that's it."

"I've pushed on with all that anger...I mean even if it's a trip to the hospital which obviously there's loads of them, I dress up. You know you'd think I was going out on some night out, you know, but I don't care."

"I've lost my friends, I am treated differently, but by wearing my make up and wearing nice clothes, it, it, it is a mask, it makes me feel better and people are nicer."

"You know I mean I put nice, really nice clothes on and I put a lot of make up on and my partner says you know, "Oh my God, you know, you look so bloody well, you don't look ill [laughs] you look fantastic and you know the doctors are going to be thinking there's nothing bloody wrong with her because you look so good", and I don't care, I want to look good now and it's because I do feel so ugly underneath. I hate my crutches, I hate wheelchairs, I hate you know having to struggle and be so oh and I hate feeling the way I do. I do feel ugly, I do feel different, and I feel people look at me different."

Attempting Suicide.

"A friend realised, what he thought I might have done and called for help. But when I tried to explain the pain, and why I'd actually done it, to the medical team I was immediately referred for psychiatric treatment, not as a pain patient that was desperate but as somebody with mental illness.

I found that to be one of the worst experiences ever. When I actually saw the psychiatrist, he asked what was wrong, I was still using the term Sudeck's atrophy then, I hadn't quite got used to the RSD or CRPS label. And as soon as I said 'Sudeck's' he asked me why I thought it wasn't a psychological problem when it, when it even sounded like 'Pseudo'.

And I can't remember whether I shouted at him first, or screamed at him, but I remember walking out and refusing ever to go back."

Some thoughts about rejection and anger

The privilege of being a carer

"I am husband and carer for Dee. Whatever I write here seems totally inadequate compared to the stories of all the sufferers of RSD. Yet the role of carer is so very important in the battle against this condition. Sadly, I fail so miserably and so often in trying to fulfil this role, but then again we are only human.

The operation that caused Dee's RSD was supposed to enable her to walk without the discomfort she had put up with for years. We were in our late 40's, early 50's in my case, Dee worked as a care assistant for the local authority, and I ran my own milk round. We have two grown up children, one wonderful granddaughter and three dogs, we were comfortable and looking forward to a period of our lives where we could enjoy all the things we had worked for. Then along came RSD! How our lives were changed!

As a husband it is heartbreaking to see Dee suffering with the pain of RSD, and to know the frustration she feels to no longer enjoy the things in her life that we took for granted, a walk through the woods with the dogs, skipping along hand in hand (like a teenager) with our granddaughter, even going to work in the morning. But wallowing in self pity gets neither of us anywhere. We had plans for the direction our lives would take us, we have had to look again at those plans and discount many of them, but in their place we have other plans, and have devised a way that we will achieve them. They may not be as grand, but they are our objectives and we are content with them. What RSD has done for us, is to bring two people who were already close, even closer. Life for us means that we have to think about what we intend to do in the context of Dee's RSD. Popping out to the shops is no longer a question of jumping in the car, it requires an element of planning, going out for a meal or to the cinema means we have to be sure that access is possible.

However whilst it is lovely to plan and achieve something together, the hum-drum nature of life continues. I have had to learn new skills. As I sit looking out of a sunny window, I have learned that the sparkles I see are not the fairies sprinkling their magic, but are in fact dust, and that same dust, when settled on a table is not an opportunity for me to write "I love you" for Dee, but needs to be wiped away. I have learned that you do finally run out of clothes to wear, and that once the cupboard is empty, there are no more plates. All these lessons were alien to me, but needed to be learned.

I have also learned that such a sweet lady (who admittedly did have her moments) can suddenly change into a screaming banshee, for no apparent reason. I have looked for the numbers '666' tattooed about her person, but have not found them yet! The mood swings she now experiences can be quite extreme, but this is part of RSD! These mood swings are upsetting for both of us, and we have had to learn to cope with them. In the early days of RSD, I became angry with myself that I had given cause for Dee to get upset, then I became angry that Dee chose to 'lose it' even though I felt that I was trying so hard. Finally we have accepted that they will happen, we will get over them, and no harm is done. Alongside this, I have moved on from a feeling of walking on eggshells whilst around Dee, where I would try to wrap her up in cotton wool, annoying her each day by asking "how are you", where she would inevitably reply "Fine" (we have our own interpretation of 'fine' provided by our daughter – "Fucked up, In pain, Neurotic, and Emotional").

Now I just raise my eyebrows, get either a thumbs up or down and the day begins. I will now argue with Dee, this may seem harsh, and I did initially find it difficult, but we both needed to understand that my life continues as well, and the fact that I said 'No' didn't mean I didn't care or that I was unwilling, it just meant 'No' and I would give my reason. I have learned to read her body language and try to step in when I feel she needs help, but without taking away her independence. I will often see her struggling with something, knowing that she will suffer later, but leave her to it. She has to have that independence, it is so important to her. Besides I can always be smug later and tell her "I told you so".

I suppose what I am trying to say in all this is to just be totally honest and truthful with each other. RSD will test any relationship, but there are benefits to come from this condition.

The path you were on may be blocked off but there are many others open to you, try them all, there will be one for you, and you can take it together.

76

I would like to share a poem 'wot I have wrote' which hopefully spells out our attitude to RSD. Feel the despair, share the helplessness, but take the positive message of:

Just Another Day

The vacuum's switched off, the duster put away,
the kitchen floor mopped, it's just another day,
I need to go to the shops to get some grub,
Time's pressing on, I can't pop into the pub.

When I married you I didn't imagine this role,
To do the manly things was my only goal,
Go out to work, provide for you and the kids,
A meal out, a holiday, watching some vids.

And changes will happen, it's out of our control,
We grow older and wiser as life takes it's toll,
We learn to adapt to whatever comes our way,
And always get through what is just another day.

But changes of this kind, though they are so rare,
Knock you for six, it just doesn't seem fair,
One day we were happy just cruising along,
Then our world falls around us, surely that is wrong.

And people around you say what will be will be,
But they don't have to fight this monster that's called RSD,
The pain you are in, they can't understand, we find,
"Just rise above it, maybe it's in your mind".

But it's not, it is real, I can see in your eyes,
And feelings of fear take me by surprise,
How could I allow someone I love so much,
To suffer this pain, to be scared of my touch.

What can I do to make this go away?
How will we get through just another day?
I've prayed to my God, and maybe he hears,
As I mumble for help through my falling tears.

So we soldier on together, a powerful team,
Nothing can halt us, 'cos we're angry and mean,
If we've lost what we had, well then so what,
So much love for each other is what we have got.

RSD you can't beat us, we are too strong,
whatever you do, we will, simply carry on,
we laugh in your face, because we will have our say,
and don't think you can stop us having another day.

So no doubts or regrets as together we live our life,
I am honoured and grateful that you are my wife,
And to all of you out there who are suffering this way,
A cure is coming, it will just take – another day!

For Dee, who I have loved from the day that I met her.

From another carer: "To be a carer or a friend of someone with Reflex Sympathetic Dystrophy or Complex Regional Pain Syndrome is almost like having the condition yourself except that you can turn the pain off when your no longer at the side of that person."

"Every waking moment is spent trying to make the day easier for that person, although that person wants to try even harder to show you that they are able to manage with their pain and carry on as normal, even if 'normal' is going to make them far worse than they would be on a good day. Sufferers want to be accepted and believed and not have to try to explain themselves away to anyone and everyone that can't often see a visible disability. Just because it's rare and no one has heard of it doesn't make it any less important than any other shitty incurable condition."

"Appointments with the General Practitioner, Nurse, Physio, Therapist and Consultants are all feared, but yet eagerly awaited in the hope that they can offer something new, something different, something that will help ease the pain, but in most cases this isn't the case and the sufferer comes away from the appointment feeling even more isolated, more helpless and thinking 'what's the point in all this'. The carer then has to put his plan into action to make the sufferer feel better, make them feel that there is hope and its worth the struggle to carry on until that day comes where someone finds the cure from a life of hell."

"This cycle continues again until the next round of appointments is due and all of the above is repeated, usually between six to twelve months."

"So what do you do in the mean time? Some sufferers are unable to work due to the severity of the condition, that's not a bad thing some might think! You ask a sufferer what they would rather be doing, sat at home, often alone, or out at work meeting people and earning a living instead of the stigma of being on benefits that isn't enough for a dog to live on."

"A carer is like a big lump of cotton wool, trying to protect the sufferer, anticipate the next bump or obstacle or blind idiot with shopping bags that thinks they have totally right of way despite the obvious discomfort shown by your companion. Even life around the house for a sufferer has its dangers for the sufferer living alone. Just feel for the person who dare not have a bath in the fear they cannot get out, or the person who cannot cook for themselves on a bad day so don't eat, or some days don't or can't get out of bed. On a good day they can get out of bed but don't get dressed or washed as they know that no one will visit, no one will call. Even the postman can't wait for you to get to the door to give you a parcel so leaves a card to tell you where to collect it from; he needn't bother because you can't get there."

"Imagine the loneliness of someone that is happy to see the dustman even if it's for a few seconds, but it is often the only contact they get when stuck inside. What adds to loneliness is the constant battle to be believed and understood by those that can make a life in hell more bearable. If anyone reading this is in any doubt what RSD/ CRPS is like give that person time to explain, they have it for life, you only need to listen for five minutes." [Barry Swallow]

What is it like being a parent seeing your child in pain?

"A parent's natural instinct is to 'make everything better.' With RSD I've learnt that actually I can do very little or nothing to help my daughter's pain. As a mother, that brings me its own kind of agony, coupled with a horrible feeling of defeat."

"Dealing with a child with RSD, I sometimes find myself 'missing' my child, as it's all too easy only to see their pain, both physical and mental. Somehow they can get lost in the pain along the way, and when I catch glimpses of the daughter I used to know, as I occasionally do, that's what brings the tears to my eyes. I really miss 'her' and there's a real grief there that makes it difficult to move on and see that this is how my daughter is now."

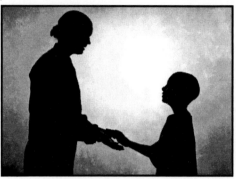

From: www.usafe.af.mil

"The pain of having a child with RSD really hits me when I see groups of her old friends, girls she grew up with, walking along in town, laughing and chatting. That can lead to a strong feeling of injustice at times. I am amazed at her capacity to cope with things that are pretty unthinkable really. I remain totally inspired and in awe of how she manages to carry on, and still laugh, despite the pain and the changes in her life because of it."

Perhaps time to smile.

"What was the matter with that one policeman?" mother asked,
after they had gone.
"Grandfather shot him," I said. "What for?" she demanded.
I told her he was a deserter.
"Of all things!" said mother.
"He was such a nice-looking young man."

In *My Life and Hard Times*, 1933
James Grover Thurber

Spreading CRPS telling us about connections in the network

For most people CRPS stays confined to the area injured, but not all. This may suggest that the basic cause does not lie in the limb itself. Here are some of many examples, where similar, but subtly different symptoms emerge. We keep dialogues and stories from now on to the briefest possible, concentrating only on emerging themes that suggest new ideas as to cause. All reports were as distressing as those presented so far. Our apologies to those whose contributions we have abbreviated.

"...a new area of RSD was caused by injuries sustained in a car accident. The new affected areas were the neck, right shoulder, arm and hand."

"And then, about a month later I started getting the pains in my left shoulder; it started travelling down into my elbow. And it was the exact same kind of pains that I had, in my right arm. Because as you get the shooting pains going down, they seem to sort of like go through your elbow and as it was going through your elbow it felt as if somebody was smacking you on the funny bone. And then after that, my left hand started closing as well."

"When the finger was eventually amputated, it went over the whole hand, sweat was pouring out of my fingers, and the finger nails grew at an alarming rate."

Another story

"That started after the operation. Well it started off on this hand, then within a couple of days it moved to my left hand then it moved to my, my left foot then the right foot. Then it went into my knee and then I experienced ripping, I become so depressed and so angry and frustrated."

Clearly CRPS can spread to other limbs, most commonly to the opposite one, but sometimes more generally.

The jumping to the other side is clearly of interest and we think an important clue to the underlying mechanism.

CRPS is not the only disease that shows this type of 'mirroring'. We see it regularly in general rheumatology, particularly in the disease rheumatoid arthritis. Dermatologists may see something similar in the skin conditions psoriasis or vitiligo.

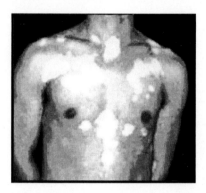

The Symmetry of Disease in Vitiligo.

Ophthalmologists see it too in a potentially blinding condition of sympathetic ophthalmitis. In this condition one eye is injured but the normal eye may respond similarly. So what is this telling us?

Let us tell you about a laboratory experiment done many years ago on an anaesthetised cat. This is not our work. A small cut was made to the nerve in the cat's leg; the aim was to study in great detail how it repaired a few days later. One of the tests involved watching the nerve sprout with an electron microscope and it did.

What baffled the investigators was far more mysterious. Scientists usually study the opposite normal side in order to see how control tissue behaves. The scientist duly dissected the exact same nerve on the other side, which had not been touched and, yes, it was sprouting in exactly the same place as the other side. Not too much and much less than the cut side. Fig 29, pg xiii.

Now isn't that remarkable? No trauma to that other leg, but the process had mirror imaged and without an electron microscope you would have seen nothing. Since then many investigators have found the same thing in a host of other disease models.

CRPS that spreads to the bowel, bladder and genitalia

You may think that since the first description of what we now call CRPS was made in the mid 1800's that if such a phenomenon was possible, health professionals would know all about it, but few do.

Surprisingly a book entitled 'CRPS, Progress in Pain Research and Management', didn't mention it. However it is briefly described in the recesses of the research world, but only tentatively. We also believe, as do others, that CRPS may start and stay in these parts and hide behind different diagnostic classifications.

Here are some further dialogues with qualitative researcher, Jenny. Dialogues we have heard many times. This is not rare in chronic CRPS of the lower limb. Men and women are affected.

"It was bizarre, what felt like a bizarre link between the bladder and the leg. At first you just think you're completely crackers."

"I just have to go to the loo when I need to, but sort of fifteen minutes I will notice an increase in that feeling coming back again. Another two minutes after that pain starts.... You get a sense of tingling and burning which increases as your bladder becomes fuller and so you get an incredible amount of pain both in your limb and your bladder and that's a sign you need to go."

"I passed urine. Well, since my accident, I was having trouble passing urine. I would have to sit on the toilet for ages and ages and concentrate, I never got off the toilet thinking my bladder's empty, it always felt really full. I had written to the Pain Society, so they sent me the address of the RSD Society. They couldn't help me about my problems with my bladder; they said they had never heard of it."

"They referred me to see an urologist and it was a lady and she said that she didn't know why I couldn't void and they did a test. I since have had bladder operations, but nothing they've done has helped me be able to void by myself. I use what they call intermittent self-catheterisation, which is not a scary thing to do... Without the catheter my bladder just builds up and builds up and there's nothing I can do about it."

"Yes, I do have a, a problem with my bowels I can't control my movements. Before I had CRPS, I never went to the toilet for days on end, that was my normal pattern, and now I often don't know when I'm going and I end up soiling myself, but I don't know if that happens to other people with this condition. It's worse in the night, when the house is quiet and you're just tired. I can pass faeces and, and not be aware of it."

"Then I had other tests done by tubes being passed into the penis and into the rectum and pressures were taken. All these signs came back relatively normal and this is when I was told then that they believe that the CRPS is in my bowel and my bladder."

The bladder, lower bowel, genitalia and foot CRPS are linked together in these dialogues, but is there a simple explanation for this distressing coupling of problems?

The feet are just short of a metre from these three organs and not neurologically linked by peripheral sensory inputs.

However, there is a simple answer within the central nervous system. Here is a picture of the answer from an old brain map produced by Prof. Wilder Penfield who established the Montreal (Canada) Neurological Institute in 1934. He placed electrodes on the conscious brain whilst operating for severe epilepsy and asked patients to report what and where they felt any response.

This cartoon character of the sensory area in the cerebral cortex has the important features drawn according to how much brain space they take up. This map is referred to as S1. Here lips and fingers with their high number of nerve endings are larger than arms and legs and the feet are beside the genitalia area. Could they be communicating with each other? The answer is yes.

There is at least one other map, called S2 in the midbrain which is more primitive than S1 and more concerned with the automatic functions of these three organs. It would seem they are linked here too.

Are there menstrual disturbances in CRPS? How does pregnancy affect CRPS? Pregnancy can precipitate CRPS in a limb as indeed breast surgery can in a hand.

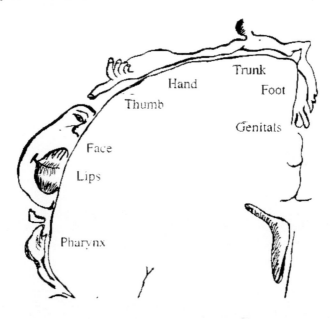

The 'Penfield map' of the sensory cortex in the upper brain, the cerebral cortex or cerebrum.

Through RSD UK and through your responses to this book we will find out more, correct the book and send the information back.

CRPS that is confined to the Bowel or Bladder

There are a variety of lower pelvic syndromes, affecting the lower bowel, bladder and sexual organs and characterised by intractable pains, that lack explanation. There are suggestions that these conditions are forms of CRPS. Indeed, we and others have seen cases where surgery to these areas for painful, sometimes trivial conditions, for example piles, has led to a considerable worsening of the pain and the development after surgery of lower limb CRPS.

Idiopathic Interstitial Cystitis, a bladder disturbance, is considered by some investigators to be a form of CRPS. The word idiopathic is used to describe a disease or disorder that has no known cause. The condition interstitial cystitis is a very disturbing disease characterized by suprapubic and pelvic pain, urinary frequency or urgency, and sterile normal urine.

Patients with IC may have the urge to void as frequently as every thirty minutes during the day and four or more times at night. Few specific and universal criteria have been established, and diagnosis is primarily a clinical one. It is grouped (by taxonomy) along with two other conditions that may have links to CRPS, urethral syndrome and prostatodynia. Fig 33.

Prostatodynia is a chronic, painful disease affecting the prostate gland. The symptoms include chills, fever, pain in the lower back and genital area, body aches, burning or painful urination, and the frequent and urgent need to urinate. The urine and fluid from the prostate reveal no evidence of a known infecting organism or of cells that the body usually produces to fight infection. These symptoms are all strikingly similar to those we see frequently in persistent CRPS that involves the lower limb.

Some obstetric conditions characterised by severe pain during sexual intercourse may also be examples. The medical word for this is dyspareunia. This leads us to 'talk dirty'.

Sex, penetration, stimulation and orgasms

"Well, I remember saying to the consultant, he says "Does anything ever help get rid of the pain…I was so embarrassed to tell him, I said yeah, orgasms help; they really help, especially if I get four or five on the trot."
"We used to end up masturbating, but it really, really helped…Yeah, trouble is, it doesn't last long. Enough… "I can't sleep, I can't sleep, the pain is just so bad and he goes "Alright then," he said, "What can help?", and I said "Well, you know, and so yeah, so we would get together and have a nice time."

"I think sexuality and the physical side to your marriage is one of the hardest things for people with CRPS to discuss. Many have said they just can't have any type of sexual relationships with their partners, and I will always say you should try this, you should try that, you know

86

because I found that, orgasms really helped me and, they make me feel more of a woman and provide me pain relief, even if it's short term. I think an hour and a half pain relief is pretty good going personally, and that's on a par with morphine."

"Well I think my physical relationship was non-existent really, initially because I just couldn't, I'd be scared that he'd bang me leg or bang me foot. So it, that, sort of the, you know, the love that we feel for one other didn't change but physically yes it did, you know that's been difficult for both of us really."

"This is a hard one you're asking because, it, it doesn't work; it hasn't worked for quite a long time. Certainly in the last two years it takes an awful lot of effort to get the penis erect, an awful lot. Usually within about ten minutes, I can no longer sustain it; bless her she's never complained, never."

"On ejaculation the pain is out of this world, I can't breathe, and I'll sit there for maybe an hour, an hour and a half even two hours trying to recover."

"Sex in the beginning was very hard, although it was just my hand that was affected. I hated any movement. So bed springs bouncing were out. In fact sex was out. I slept with my hand on a chair beside the bed.

Eventually we realised we could not go on like this. We both missed the closeness so we made love very slowly, with my hand on the chair - not very romantic, but we did it. I tried not to cause much movement or vibrations. Eventually things improved over the years. Nobody tell you about these things."

"When the RSD got worse and went to all my limbs, it was hard. It is painful and awkward. It is a case of finding a position that is suitable, and where to put the legs and hands. We joke about getting a horse hoist to hang from the ceiling for when things get too bad. You can just picture it!"

"Now I have RSD internally I find it very awkward. Hubby doesn't know, but I don't always have any feeling. Also as I also have bladder problems. I worry I might wet myself now. That along with the pain stops me relaxing, and when I do climax, the pain shoots up to my head and I get a really bad head. The pain internally is awful."

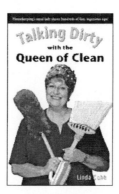

Talking about sex for doctors, patients and carers can be tricky.
From www.simonsays.com.

"When my symptoms started I was in an extremely unhappy and often violent and verbally abusive marriage and any type of sexual interaction was rare. When my 'new' relationship started I was terrified and in pain. Trust and understanding was the key. A few years ago I was diagnosed as having 'meraglia parasthetica' [an example of an entrapment neuropathy] in the right side; the only way I could describe the pain back then was like having an orgasm in my leg, but so big it is painful. But, as the relationship blossomed and trust grew I found this could be a bit of a bonus; an impending orgasm increased the pleasant sensation in the leg, but not the pain, it took the emphasis away from the RSD pain onto the leg sensations."

Similar stories are told us by amputees, or to be more precise lower limb amputees, without any history of CRPS and meeting none of the diagnostic criteria for it.

Mrs S had an amputation many years ago and was recently married. "Congratulations on your marriage Anne", I say in clinic by way of an introduction. Yes I'm sometimes pleasant!

"Thank you", she replies and stops. I wait without interruption.

"I know it's nothing to do with you but I'm having terrible pain during sex."

"In your stump?" I ask looking at her steadily.

She averts her eyes, "Well yes, but that's not the problem. Its deep in my vagina…and the gynaecologist says I'm fine…..and I am going to see a psychiatrist… in case I am mad."

"And are you?"

She replies, "… probably not."

We find here of a variety of profoundly different stories. Some patients find sex and orgasms intolerable; for others it causes momentary relief, for many it has sedative qualities, and for others problems with relationships. All are explicable to some extent. The particular interest is those that find it brings relief. It is easy to understand the opposite by reference to the sensory map S1 or S2, where we would explain it by sensory spreading in the brain, which we know occurs. It is more difficult to explain the opposite unless you argue it is mere distraction, a moment where pain is not attended to. But what is this phenomenon? It leads to a far more complex question; can you feel, or attend to, two pains at once? This leads to another question; what is attention?

Here is a simple experiment. You are asked to attend to a problem, say counting backwards, and then we apply a painful heat stimulus. Will you feel the pain as much as when you just had the heat without the stimulus? No! For an identical heat stimulus you report less pain when your mind is diverted. Could you feel two pains simultaneously? We believe not, but you can switch your attention rapidly between them unless one is totally dominating. Therefore you can describe two pains, which is not the same as feeling them together. An orgasm, or better multiple orgasms, is obviously dominating, but for some the pain always dominates and proper sex is impossible.

For most women complete sexual pleasure comes from clitoral stimulation and not vaginal penetration, though in some it is both. Vaginal penetration may be painful in CRPS and this occurs, we believe, more commonly than clitoral pain which in some at least seems immune from the problem. A female orgasm involves different brain areas from a male climax.

There are considerable differences between the male and female brain and one important area is in the midbrain, the hypothalamus, which controls many autonomic activities and the hippocampus. We talk about these two areas later but this is where they are.

The hypothalamus and hippocampus

Men have difficulties and conflicting stories to tell. For some, penile stimulation causes pain. For others the pain induces variable impotence. Some of the prescribed medication can cause impotence. Some find orgasms render them pain-free and others it worsens; some like the women can experience an orgasm feeling in the limb affected which may be pleasant or unpleasant.

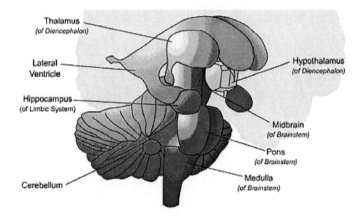

The hypothalamus in the midbrain controls many functions including hunger, thirst, pain, pleasure and the sex drive.
The hippocampus controls memories dreams and helps us determine here we are it is sex hormone sensitive.

From www.webschoolsolutions.com.

The solution to sexual problems is the same in CRPS as any other state - talk about it.

Which is not easy, and why we wrote about it

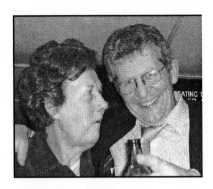

Mr Don Foster (MP Bath LIB-DEM) 'talking about it', allegedly, to an author's friend, Jean, who 'doesn't do bedroom talk'.

Photographer David Blake

Phantoms, pain and swelling

A phantom is something that can be seen or heard or whose presence can be felt, but that is not physically present. Phantom pains and sensations were first described in amputees and initially they were not believed. We provide some 'quotes from the Web' to demonstrate their reality and their remarkable similarity to CRPS sensations.

"Despite its 'ghostly' connotation, phantom sensation is most certainly a realistic, tangible event experienced by millions of amputees world-wide."

"Phantom sensation is usually experienced by most amputees at one time or another. Phantom sensation is not just the feeling of having a limb when no limb is present (which usually goes away). It is a term used for any sensation or pain originating from a residual (stump) limb. Phantom sensation can range from tingling sensations to severe, sharp, stabbing pain that can only be controlled via professional pain management."

"Phantom pain comes on strong with sharp, shooting pains originating in the bottom of the residual limb and experienced in the 'missing' shin or knee or foot area. The sensation for me is like an electric shock of pain or a sharp stabbing feeling. The pain can come on fast or slow and have a wide range of intensity. The pain may last a few hours or a few days and longer. Phantom sensation feels like tingling or pins and needles in the stump end. It is very similar your foot falling asleep and it feels sort of numb and tingly for a minute or two; except phantom sensation can go on for days. I've had this feeling for up to five days in a row, resulting in lack of sleep, edginess and ending up in a full-blown attack of pain."

Phantom swelling in CRPS

"You feel as if your foot is swollen even though it's not swollen".

"It (the hand) feels massive, it feels massive."

"The leg feels a lot larger than what it is. It's easily twice, three times the size of a normal leg."

There are two kinds of swelling in this last dialogue, one obvious to the patient and observer, another not. The first is recognised by the classification system we discussed, the other isn't. They are of course equally real, to the sufferer. The non-observable one comes with more distress, as we discussed. We refer to the non-observable as phantom; not imaginary, fabricated or hysterical. Others with less clinical experience do not. This is a major source of litigation difficulties, not to mention frustration.

The observable is oedema fluid. This is spelt edema in American English. It is caused by leakage of protein and water through altered blood vessels. Endothelial cells line blood vessels and they separate as the blood vessel wall relaxes. Usually this is most obvious in the acute phases. Swelling often settles later, but may come and go.

The hand and feet, having large sensory, inputs usually suffer phantom sensations more; it may extend to a whole limb. Remember the hand and face lie close together in the brain map, perhaps explaining why the areas seem to fuse or merge in the lady with the 'out-of-body' type experience.

The word 'phantom' was used to describe these 'ghosts' as the limb did not exist, but patients certainly experienced them and pain was a common accompaniment. Previous pains in the limb clearly affect the nature of the pain. This suggests we hold pain memories, and studies suggest that sensory inputs of sufficient intensity, and for an adequate period, may produce lasting changes in central neural structures. These

92

affect the 'cognitive-evaluative' systems we have described often giving them characteristics that are very distressing.

Simple memories and stimuli can then generate responses as we find in CRPS. Limbs may be remembered in awkward postures, arthritis recalled, stiffness and swelling feelings may be generated. Now we consider more phantoms in CRPS. Consider this possibility though that all the sensations may be retained knowledge and the experience of them triggered by the same kind of non-noxious stimuli that trigger allodynia.

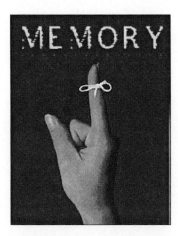

Some pains are pains recalled from
Previous exposure 'pain memories'
www.exploratorium.edu.

More apparitions, ghouls and ghosts

Where are my limbs?

"I have feelings of panic about the left arm, not just the chance of it being touched by someone but the fact that I really cannot locate it unless I can see it. I wake in the night in a panic thinking I have lost my arm. If I am working I keep looking at it constantly to feel reassurance; depending on what I am doing that arm could feel anywhere between on my body and a few feet away – I find this incredibly difficult to describe, it is also frightening!"

"...but one of the nasty ones is I can't always tell where both legs are, it most often happens when I am sat with my legs under a table. Both legs feel numb yet I can feel them; if I stand on something such as a bottle cap I can't feel it is there, I check my feet regularly. If someone were to touch one of my feet I really could not tell which one was being touched unless I was watching; I feel very frightened about this."

"When I am stacking boxes, small ones, at work I topple over to the right hand side, every time. Triangular boxes are the worst. Bags with stripes on – we don't use those any more in the shop as they did similar things to the buildings, they moved, I swear they really bloody well moved!"

"When I wake up the left hand always feels as though it is on my face, regardless of where it really is. I first mentioned this to a doctor in September 2000 and I was ridiculed badly, so much so I left the clinic."

These phenomena may be similar to some 'out-of-body' experiences. During an out-of-body experience you seem to be awake and to see your body and the world from a location outside the physical body.

A closely related experience is autoscopy, which is characterized by the experience of seeing one's body outside of you. These phenomena have been recently researched by Olaf Blanke, a Swiss neurologist. This is what he concluded. The jargon is complex but the meaning clear.

"We suggest that out of body experiences and autoscopy are related to a failure to integrate proprioceptive, tactile and visual information with respect to one's own body (disintegration in personal space) and by a vestibular dysfunction leading to an additional disintegration between personal (vestibular) space and extra personal (visual) space. We argue that both disintegrations (personal and personal–extra personal) are necessary for the occurrence of out of body experiences and AS, and that they are due to a paroxysmal cerebral dysfunction of the tempero-parietal junction in a state of partially and briefly impaired consciousness."

In other words something disturbs another complex network at more than one point.

94

Strange experiences of this kind come about by disintegration of brain networks that involve the ear and associated organs (vestibular), the eyes and an area of the cerebral hemisphere, the tempero-parietal junction. The experiments done here were on epileptics who had such symptoms associated with brain discharges.

In the cases above, where the experience was local and not general, lines and shapes integrated by visual–vestibular circuits in the lower brain seem to set off a further disintegration of the network and cause pain and movement problems in discreet areas.

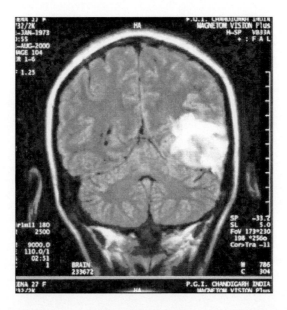

The tempero-parietal area is the white bit. This is an abnormal NMR scan of a stroke victim.

Professor Olaf Blanke used NMR imaging to see these areas, but our patients' stories alone suggest this anatomical distribution for at least some of the pain network. We get more anatomical clues from other strange symptoms where we embrace the concept of 'synesthesia'. This would be another way to interpret some of the ghouls described above.

Don't Touch My Good Side Either; Synchiria

Mrs. Smith "May we touch you good foot… thank you… where did you feel it?"

"Odd… in both my good and bad foot. In the bad it hurt"

This is an example of what has been called **synchiria** in which a stimulus applied to one side of the body is referred to both sides. Here simple touch is transferred to the other and causes pain. We and others call this dysynchiria.

The same thing happens in amputees where the sensation is transferred to the phantom. This phenomenon suggests precise connections between perceptual responses in both sides of the brain. In dysinchiria it creates an impulse in an area linked to the dysfunctional pain network, hence pain.

This provides another mechanism for the disease switching side but it is confusing to most sufferers. It is our experiences that touch from strangers are more likely to elicit this than self-touch. The key observation is the precise mapping of the 'synchiria' phenomenon. The symmetry is precise and input specific, so light touch is felt on the other side as light touch and pain as pain.

Whilst words and definitions of words are crucial to science and its progress you will be noticing that different words are used to describe similar phenomena. We return to this overlap as we discuss allodynia again in more detail.

Strange Sweating

Perspiration, or sweat, is the body's way of cooling, whether that extra heat comes from exercise or from over-stimulated nerves. Nerve cells from the sympathetic nervous system connect to the sweat glands. There are two types of sweat glands: eccrine - the most numerous kind is found all over the body, particularly on the palms of the hands, soles of the feet and forehead and apocrine - mostly confined to the armpits (axilla) and the anal-genital area. There is a rich blood supply to sweat glands which are enclosed by a complex array of nerves of different kinds: Both autonomic and pain-sensitive nerves are present.

Sweat glands typically end in hair follicles rather than pores. As we mentioned, sweating responds to your emotional state. So, when you are nervous, anxious or afraid, there is an increase in sympathetic nerve activity in your body as well as an increase in epinephrine secretion from your adrenal gland. These substances act on your sweat glands, particularly those on the palms of your hand and your armpits, to make sweat. Thus, you feel a 'cold' sweat. Also, the increased sympathetic nerve activity in the skin changes its electrical resistance, which is the basis of the galvanic skin response used in lie detector tests. When sweat evaporates from the surface of your skin, it removes excess heat and cools you. Excessive sweating is called diaphoresis or hyperhidrosis.

Localised over-activity of the sympathetic nervous system in CRPS, a cause of pain and caused by pain and emotion, creates the local sweating. It is confined to the CRPS area, but some patients, indeed many, get night sweats that are generalised. In patients with hand involvement it may also involve the face on that side.

"Basically, if something's made me jump, say you've got a one of the children come in and shout, 'Boo' really loud and it startles me, that arm will start sweating."

"If it gets sweaty for any reason, it doesn't alter the pain but it alters the way it actually feels. My hands are shiny with this condition and if I was to hold anything or put my hand on, or anything where you could see the sweat coming up, it just perspires my hands, my feet, underneath my right armpit. As I'm talking to you now it's burning under there and soaking at the same time."

"In the, in the evening it gets worse…"

The first description would seem to fit a description of 'allodynic sweating'. This is an example of a pathological sweating reaction caused by localised sympathetic over-activity to a simple non-noxious stimulus. There is another explanation albeit more complicated. It relates to how sensations and perceptions can become muddled.

Synaesthesia

The scientific word for this is 'synaesthesia' or 'synesthesia' and means, 'joined sensation' and here is a definition from the web.

"Synesthesia (Greek, syn = together + aisthesis = perception) is the involuntary physical experience of a cross-modal association. That is, the stimulation of one perceptual modality reliably causes a perception in one or more different senses."

People will describe the colour green as having a taste and certain alphabetic letters seem linked to colour. Some taste shapes. How common synesthesia is in CRPS we do not know. Nor do we know if synesthesia can come before the commoner features of CRPS. Normal people have synesthetic experiences. They do not, as far as we know, embrace pain perceptions crossed to other perceptions.

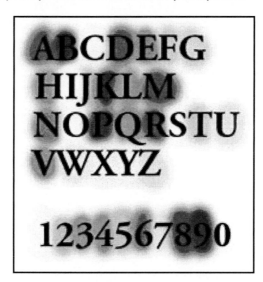

One in every 2500 people share this unique joined sensory experience
From www.thesheridanreporter.com

Some scientists maintain that all of us begin our lives as synaesthetes until we start to separate our senses. Experimental observation of human newborns suggests that a spatial link exists between vision and auditory systems in the prenatal brain. Clearly, if correct, most of us outgrow the synesthesia and learn to differentiate different perceptions discretely. This would prevent sensory overload, but its emergence in our patients clearly causes overload. The hippocampus in the lower brain is critical for this experience. The hippocampus we have briefly mentioned and we will do so again.

So should we be describing some of these strange phenomena as 'synesthetic' perceptions rather than phantoms?

In synesthesia one sensation translates to another response. Coming next are a bunch of other responses set off by another stimulus.

Movement, spasm and shakes

"...because my hand's sort of like closed up and I can't straighten my arm...they're trying to sort of like really push the treatment to get my arm straightened and open my hand and things like that. But my body's reacting to that. If you stress me mentally or physically it closes"

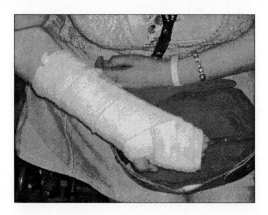

Splinting a hand with trophic changes and there is our Charity's bracelet again.
"My hand sort of like curls under and it's as if all your muscles in your arm's just sort of like reacting to many things and just really going tense."

"Sometimes they're locked you know like you can spread your fingers, I can a bit today, but other times they are like that and they're rigid and there's no way I can move them whatever. Lots of things cause this."

"I was half way down the stairs with both my sticks and leg went into spasm and when it goes into spasm or a multiple spasm it shouts right through your body and because my knees locked the spasm is shooting against a locked area, so the pain is even worse than what it would normally be. I leant forward, next thing I knew I was at the bottom of the stairs."

Hands and feet that turn in and claw, locking, shaking, lack of movement, weakness, hiding the limb from sight (theirs) are all linked either directly to another stimulus. You could say the network is super-charged and an input anywhere causes another output in the periphery, perhaps a form of synesthesia, but not one embraced by the present definition.

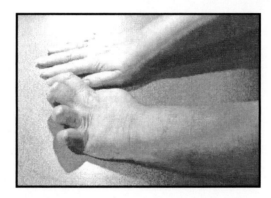

Locked and clawed for a short time. See also Fig. 34 pg xiv

It occurs after emotional stress or a small bump elsewhere. Here may be a legal case of this kind of thing that mattered.

Frank's been involved in a medico-legal dispute. The extent of his handicap is disputed on the grounds that they have proof conclusive that he can sometimes do things he says he can't. His injury was in part due to failure of his employers to maintain normal safety standards.

Frank had seen his medico-legal examiner who found a considerable decrease in movement and surmised that this was 'a disability' and could reasonably be considered to cause significant 'handicap'. Frank had been touched and prodded and his hand had gone into spasm. The doctor described Frank's significant handicap in his report.

100

On the next day Frank visits a supermarket with his wife. The boredom of staying at home all day 'gets to him'. She asks him to get a can from the shelf and he clearly moves his affected hand which is no longer in spasm. What Frank did not know, until some time later, was that behind him was a man with a briefcase. Indeed it contained his work, a surveillance camera, as requested by his employer's lawyer. Frank's solicitor was convinced Frank was overstating his problem or a liar.

Frank was distraught and as the solicitor told him what had been seen Frank's hand shook and then would not move. Frank abandoned his claim and he has not worked since. He sees a psychologist for counselling.

"Honest Abe" from Odds and Ends.
Robert Crumb

Neglect and alienation

We turn now to disgust and neglect-like feelings. Disgust is easier to understand. A CRPS limb may well be unattractive for the sufferer, but neglect, alienation and depersonalisation are different and occur commonly in CRPS.

Carefully study how people describe their limbs in these dialogues which we have shortened.

"I feel that when it looks bad I feel repulsed by it then I automatically assume that other people will be."

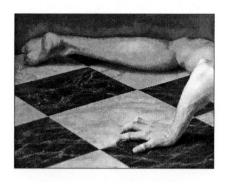

Neglect and alien type limb problems seem common in CRPS
"Element of alienation."
from jan@janesmann.com

"I feel disgust, I know it sounds a very strong word to use but I'm disgusted that my arm is this way. It is a withered, useless item which has let me and the ones I love, down"

"I felt almost repulsed by it. I didn't want anything to do with it."

"I sit there talking to it. The hand to me is nothing."

"Now I said, "chop it off, get rid of it, I don't want it."

When we talk of our limbs they are part of us. They live in our space. Our space is called 'egocentric space'. The space around us is called 'allocentric space'.

We call our limbs 'my arm, my hand'. We don't call it 'it' or 'the arm.' In the dialogues above the limbs are in the impersonal tense. In order to understand why these patients have switched from the personal to the impersonal we need to understand how we know ourselves and how we know we are all joined up correctly in our world of 'self and me.'

The internal representation of space involves the integration of different sensory inputs. These come from our nerves taking readings from all over our skeletal muscles. The muscles, ligaments and joints all send messages via the specialised 'proprioceptive' nerves. These are a branch of sensory nerves, ending in muscles, tendons, and joints, that provide a sense of the body's position. They respond to stimuli from within the body. For example, you can tell where your arm is, blindfolded. They are linked to the eyes and the vestibular system of the ears. One purpose of the vestibular system is to help you locate the position and motion of your head in space either during rotation or along a line. The vestibular system is divided into two receptor organs to accomplish these two tasks. The canals link to your eyes to keep them still in space while your head moves around them.

We took one patient with CRPS and an amputated leg and stirred up her ear, and therefore her vestibular system, by dripping cold water into the ear canal. She responded with more pain and a host of other symptoms.

Similar experiments have been done in patients after a stroke of the parietal region of the brain. These patients have visual symptoms and are unaware of the one side of a room. However, put water in an ear and they can see it. Some patients with this specific stroke don't recognise half of themselves even though they can see themselves normally. This is referred to as parietal neglect and the loss of knowledge of ones own body space is called '**anosognosia**'.

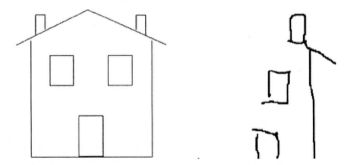

A stroke has affected the parietal lobe of the brain. The patient is trying to draw the house but misses the left side out. This is visual neglect. Patients with CRPS don't do this but can have other neglect problems similar to anosognosia. They are often subtle and the patient may be unaware of it.

Some with severe strokes may be unaware that anything is wrong, just that one half of their body isn't theirs, but they don't mind. Others can show hostile 'alien type hatred reactions' similar to those described here. There are other apparently 'normal' people with an overwhelming desire to amputate a limb as it feels completely foreign. This is known as 'body integrity identity disorder' or '**apotemnophilia**'.

All these processes are driven by the brain and all appear to have differently located lesions disrupting the normal representation of self in space. Here are dialogues with CRPS patients.

"I'm always walking into the side of doors."

"My wife is clumsy she keeps putting her wheelchair into the door frame."

Are they just clumsy or do they have difficulties in relating their egocentric space to their allcentric space? We accept that scientific language can sound daft but we hope you see the difference between these two states. One is not a problem the other is.

CRPS sufferers can divide a line in half with a pencil; some parietal stroke patients go off to one side. Are sounds neglected on one side? We do not know. There are serious spatial awareness problems however. We discuss others later; like buildings jumping. These dialogues are different.

"But bits of me are missing".

"If someone said "where's your right arm?" you know vaguely because of where it touches but it's almost like gone semi-translucent, it's almost not visible, up here. (Points to head)"

"Like if I try and picture my body and my arm they're there's no forearm at all; the hand, there are no fingers, there is a palm but it doesn't know really how to connect to my elbow at all."

"I was losing visual recognition of the whole of my hand; you know I've said I still can't see any fingers".

"The hand didn't have any fingers, it was quite fuzzy."

"The whole arm was almost disappearing and it feels as if it's a great distance from the wrist to the elbow."

"There's nothing there at all that I can actually see the floor. I can see a big toe and I can't see anything else from my knee down, there's nothing there at all."

Some CRPS patients don't seem recognise themselves intact yet amputees consider they are, or nearly, when they are not. Here is a picture of what a phantom amputee feels they have recreated by a graphic artist using a computer reconstruction.

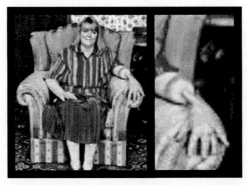

An Amputee with a phantom arm. Look carefully at her left arm this is how she feels it.

It shows some similarities and some large differences to the descriptions we have given. The explanation seems to lie in the Penfield brain map S1 we showed earlier. The area between the wrist and the hand has little spatial representation on the map and doesn't seem to get much phantom attention; indeed it seems regularly neglected in CRPS. However many patients say different things, like fingers merging or blending or separating or vanishing. This, we believe is due to one area taking up so much space that it squeezes the adjoining area and removes your sense of awareness. This may sound unlikely, but imaging studies clearly show that this may happen. If an area of the brain is overloaded with inputs it expands and if underused the adjoining area may encroach into it.

The final straw; perception overload

We have discussed pain perceptions in detail, particularly the excessive pain reactions to normal or slightly painful stimuli. The emotive nature of these dialogues can seem extreme and suggests to health professionals and others that they are exaggerated and thereby fabricated. It is clear that this rarely is the case and CRPS patients resent the implications and others' responses add to the burden of this disease. Most of us are aware that "If you add to the truth, you subtract from it." This is a quote from the Talmud (דומלת) which is a record of rabbinic deliberations on Jewish law, ethics, customs, legends and stories with an interesting print layout.

Pain is only one problem that is generated from a noxious insult. Over time other perceptual problems become manifest, and in this section we give examples of some to demonstrate just how confusing this disease may be to some.

We have five main senses: sight, smell, taste, hearing and touch. Each of these senses detects a feature of the environment and generates nerve signals to carry this information to the brain. Together they allow us to see the world in a similar fashion and believe it to be ordered and us sane. When things go wrong we, and others, believe that we are insane. We illustrate this with examples of the strange world inhabited by CRPS sufferers,

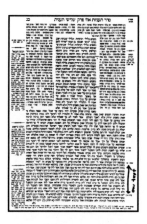

Hebrew text from the Talmud
From www.etzchayim.org/rabbi.

many of which are not vocalised. However down in the depths of our laboratories we can extract it!

Touch and Agnosia

Here is an experiment we asked a CRPS sufferer patient to do over the Web. She has CRPS of the right hand.

"I told Lee and Kirsty about the experiment you wanted me to do. They got five items each and put each item in a separate carrier bag. They took it in turns to let me reach in to a plastic bag - first with my left hand then with my right.

I had no idea what to expect, what I got was not what I expected and this has thrown me."

Actual OBJECT	Right NORMAL	Left CRPS
Brush	Brush	Keys
Badge	Badge	Keys
Diary	Diary	No idea
Scissors	Scissors	Pens
Yo –Yo	Yo –Yo	Credit card
Cards	Cards	No idea
Diablo string	Diablo string	No idea

"On the ones I got wrong, I don't think I got wrong because of what I was feeling or responding to touch, it felt as though (not sure I can explain this) that I knew what it was, but couldn't find the right word for the objects. With the left hand I was searching for the right word to use. When I said what I thought the objects were I knew I was wrong but didn't know how or why I said the word I had said. No problems with the right hand at all, I said them all as soon as I felt the objects. Not a pleasant experience overall but please let me know if this is what you anticipated. Happy to help, David."
This is what a colleague of ours, a neurologist of distinction, concluded.

"This is an 'agnosia syndrome,' or more precisely an example of asterioagnosia, and suggestive of a non-dominant parietal lesion in the cerebrum."

This is correct except it's not caused by what he is more familiar with, a stroke or a tumour, but created by an enhanced CNS electrical discharge, itself generated by the threat of putting the CRPS hand into a bag? That, by the way, was a hypothesis and not a statement of fact. To test the 'threat hypothesis' we would need to desensitise her to the threat and repeat the experiment many times. Wait for the next edition.

Let's talk a little more about the parietal lobe and agnosia, which simply means a failure to recognise. Here is a definition from the web.

Agnosia is a rare disorder characterized by an inability to recognize and identify objects or persons despite having knowledge of the characteristics of the objects or persons. People with agnosia may have difficulty recognizing the geometric features of an object or face, or may be able to perceive the geometric features but not know what the object is used for or whether a face is familiar or not. Agnosia can be limited to one sensory modality such as vision or hearing. For example, a person may have difficulty in recognizing an object as a cup or identifying a sound as a cough. Agnosia can result from strokes, dementia, or other neurological disorders. It typically results from damage to specific brain areas in the occipital or parietal lobes of the brain. People with agnosia may retain their cognitive abilities in other areas.

Our patient then has touch agnosia, and another problem, as she knows she is giving a wrong answer. You could therefore call this dysnosia, suggesting a degree of recognition that cannot be processed fully. There is no word dysnosia in the dictionary. There is however a word called dystonia which is a big feature of CRPS.

Dystonia

Dystonia is a disorder characterized by muscle contractions, which force certain parts of the body into abnormal, sometimes painful, movements or postures, which occur even if you don't want them to. Movement is a very complicated process and involves many areas in the brain.

Musicians, darts players and computer board operators may suffer from dystonia. The common underlying factor seems to be the constant stimulation of a small area in the periphery. In darts players the thumb and index finger have been shown to fuse when looked at by magnetic imaging. There is a smaller distance between the representations of the digits in somatosensory cortex for the affected hand of dystonic musicians than for the hands of normal people. The same thing happens in CRPS; digits fuse and take up a greater area. Here it is not caused by repeated movement causing nerve firing, but pain doing the same thing.

Dystonia is managed by neurologists primarily and, like many other chronic neurological disorders, was recognized as a distinct entity only relatively recently. Even before the term 'dystonia' was coined, people with the syndrome were being reported explicitly in the literature.

In 1911, Hermann Oppenheim, a Berlin neurologist who wrote a leading textbook of neurology, was impressed with the variation in muscle tone seen in a neurological syndrome that he had seen in young boys. He invented the term 'dystonia' to indicate that muscle tone was hypotonic on one occasion and in tonic muscle spasm at another. [Meaning the tone of the muscles fluctuated between too much and too little.] This was usually, but not exclusively, elicited upon movements exercised at will.

Dystonia also caused twisted postures associated with the muscle spasms affecting limbs. It occurs regularly in CRPS it can come and go and threat can worsen it rapidly. In CRPS reflexes may be pathologically brisk or abnormal (e.g. Babinski reflex) and may suggest to doctors a structural cord injury or brain tumour when there is none. Muscles may contract and relax very fast, this is called clonus. It is a feature of dystonia and we see it regularly in CRPS.

Investigators believe that the dystonias result from an abnormality in a variety of areas of the brain including the basal ganglia where some of the messages that initiate muscle contractions are processed. It is inherited in some and the gene has been identified.

Not everyone carrying the gene has the disease. Clearly other factors, possibly other genes, are needed for the disease to be expressed.

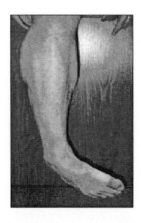 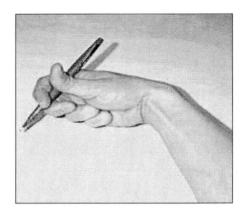

Dystonia: note how similar this is to the pictures of some CRPS legs and hands in CRPS.

A few more words on the parietal lobe and strange perceptions

The parietal lobes can be divided into two functional regions. One involves sensation in and perception out and the other is concerned with integrating (linking) sensory inputs say touch, with vision.

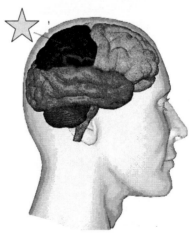

The Parietal lobe

The first function joins together sensory information to form a single perception. The second function constructs a 'spatial coordinate system'. This means it helps us represent and interpret the world around us. Or to put it even more simply; we can see the leaves and the trees. We can see the eyes within the face.

Individuals with damage to the parietal lobes may show striking deficits, such as abnormalities in body image and spatial relations and we have seen examples of both in CRPS. Here is another problem some get. Look carefully at this image.

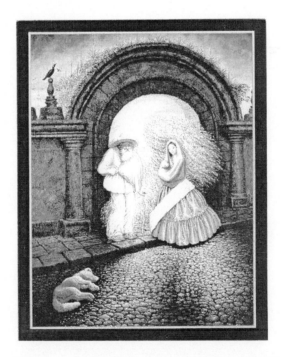

Can you see the face and the people inside it?

Some CRPS suffers find this confusing and disquieting; others do not see the girl or the old man even when pointed out to them. This may represent an example of simultanagnosia, which is described below. To see neither is rare in normal people. Here they are.

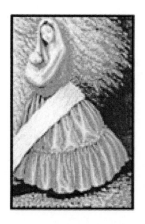 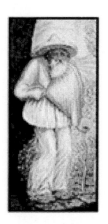

Damage to the left parietal lobe can result in what is called 'Gerstmann's Syndrome'. It includes right-left confusion, difficulty with writing (**agraphia**) and difficulty with mathematics (**acalculia**). It can also produce disorders of language (**aphasia**) and the inability to perceive objects normally (**agnosia**).

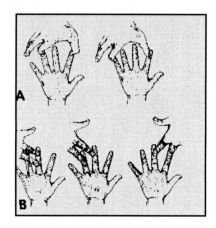

With your eyes closed which fingers am I touching?
Tests like this are difficult for some.

Damage to the right parietal lobe can result in neglecting part of the body or space (**contra-lateral neglect**), which can impair many self-care skills such as dressing and washing. Right side damage can also cause difficulty in making things (constructional **apraxia**), denial of deficits (**anosagnosia**) and drawing ability.

Damage or dysfunction on both sides can cause 'Balint's syndrome', a visual attention and motor syndrome. This is characterized by the inability to voluntarily control the gaze (ocular **apraxia**), inability to integrate components of a visual scene (**simultanagnosia**), and the inability to accurately reach for an object with visual guidance (optic **ataxia**). We have not seen much of this in CRPS apart from simultanagnosia, but we have not tested fully yet. We have listed these parietal dysfunctional problems in full hoping you will write to us if you can relate them to any difficulties you have. Thank you.

Our patients' descriptions do indeed suggest abnormal discharges in both parietal lobes perhaps more on the right. We have discussed 'neglect like phenomena' which suggests the right side, and forms of agnosia, difficulty perceiving objects, suggesting the left. Simultanagnosia suggests both sides. All are partial and change with time and are not identical to the forms that occur with strokes or other brain problems.

In our test of perception with the hand in the bag we have tested the ability of a CRPS hand to interact with its environment without visual clues and then interpret it. It is clearly faulty, but not so when vision assists. There is a problem of spatial perception and three areas of the brain are involved in this. One we have already mentioned is the parietal cortex. Another is the pre-frontal cortex and finally the hippocampus which is an odd shape and is tucked lower down. Here is a picture of these areas.

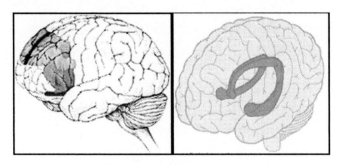

From Brain connection.com

113

The prefrontal cortex (left) is central to organizing the distributed information contained in the nervous system. The hippocampus (right) is involved in linking information systems from the eye, ear and body, helping with memory, creating dreams.

These systems are linked to the pain network.

Problems with spatial awareness

Here we perform another study of spatial awareness. Look at this for thirty seconds.

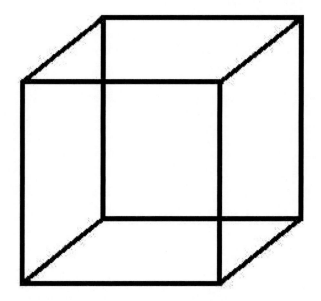

It is a Necker cube, an example of an ambiguous figure.

This is a simple two-dimensional line drawing of a cube that we see as three-dimensional. You will find it is unstable, if you look at it hard it will flick and keep flicking. You see two possible orientations. How fast it flicks varies from person to person and over time. For some it never flicks.

All responses are normal, but the dialogue below is most unusual. For this CRPS patient, staring at the cube did the strangest things.

"The first few seconds of the test made my eyes feel very strange and a sort of pressure feeling inside my head. The cube was flicking very fast at some points and I felt dizzy, nauseous and very strange, but the pressure feeling got worse as the minute wore on. My head was jiggling about and I couldn't stop. It was a good ten minutes after doing the test before I wanted to look at anything."

Another reported this: even stranger.
"It's flicking very fast. My arm has 'moved' to beside my ear. My hand is next to my head. It made me feel surreal. The arm feels as if it is not on my elbow; like it has broken into pieces… this is not nice."

Other linked and strange things

"Traffic cones send me dippy when they are on both sides (such as motorway works) and the left arm always throbs, I have always put this throbbing down to putting the left hand on the steering wheel for driving through cones etc, left hand is normally on my knee as I steer one-handed."

Here is a letter we received in response to this request. "Tell us if you have strange feelings or unusual problems we have not asked about."

"Yes, using the wrong words without realising I have done and then arguing because I think they heard me wrong: A typical one at work, in the shop, is:

Me, "Can you pass me the till?"
Kay, "The what?"
Me "The till."
Kay, "Do you mean the price gun?"

Here is another different example; at home.

Me "Can you feed the table?"
Kay "Do you mean the dog?"
Me "That's what I said."

When the RSD gets worse the dog notices a very nasty sweet smell that smells 'like death'. I can smell it."

"My leg smells."

To our knowledge this has not been described before though some patients have reported to us a hypersensitivity to smell. Occasionally normal tastes seem unpleasant. Here are some great stories sent to RSD UK. Thanks for these.

Smell, dogs and CRPS

"Since complaining about the pains in my knee after my accident, all dogs that I have known for a few years, plus new dogs that I have met since starting with this condition, have really amazed me. My mother and father-in-law have a small whippet dog, called Bambi, who before my injury would visit and she would come to both sides of me. She would cuddle up against either my right or left knee, all depending on how she was feeling.

Since I have been complaining of pain these last few months and particularly the fear of anyone coming near my knee, the dog has changed.

She will now sit on the right side, but a distance away from the leg. She will try and sniff the knee but without touching it and backs away and guards my comfort zone. If anyone is walking towards my bad side, she stands up on all four paws and growls at the person. This is clever because if a person goes to pass me on my good side, she does not move. Great dog."

"My friend has a Rottweiller, called Heidi, that I have often looked after. Before the injury the dog used to try and sit on the knee of either me or my husband. Without touching the knee, she now seems drawn to sniff at the knee, and will not sit at my bad side, especially if she has just tried sniffing the knee. She will get up and move to the left. She does not sit on my knee now."

"I went to stay a couple of nights; with a friend who has a Jack Russell called Jess and here she is below.

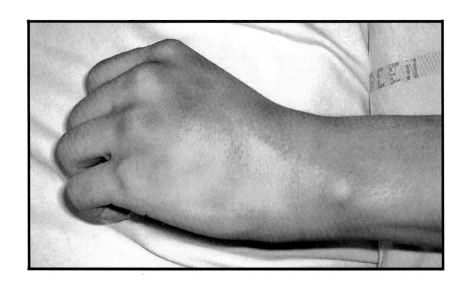

[Fig 1] Above: The worst pain imaginable, allodynia in CRPS (page 13)

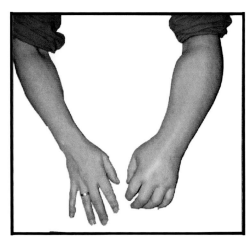

[Fig 2]   Above: Complex Regional Pain Syndrome (CRPS), also known as   Reflex Sympathetic Dystrophy (RSD) (page 13)

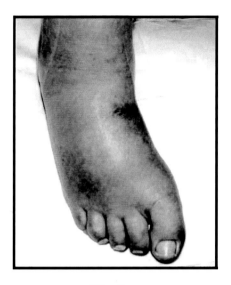

[Fig 3]

Above: Complex Regional Pain Syndrome (CRPS), also known as Reflex Sympathetic Dystrophy (RSD) (page 13)

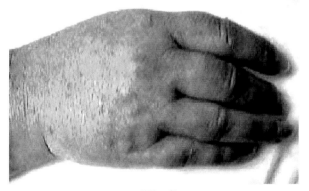

[Fig 4]

Clawing of the hand "like a hook". This sign, shown in a mild form here, may come and go (page 20)

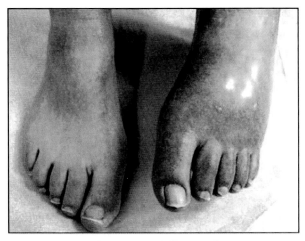

[Fig 5] Classical early CRPS is often easy to reverse with repeated desensitization and graded exercises. (page 25)

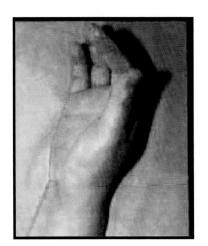 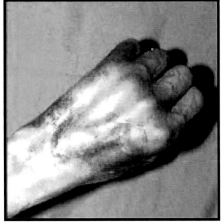

[Figs 6 – 7, above & 8 overleaf]

Three CRPS patients - but they have very different symptoms and signs. Some look completely normal at first glance (page 28)

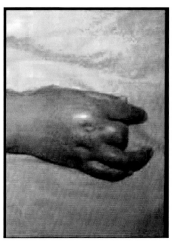

[Fig 8 above, Figs 6 & 7 previous page]

Three CRPS patients - but they have very different symptoms and signs. Some look completely normal at first glance (page 28)

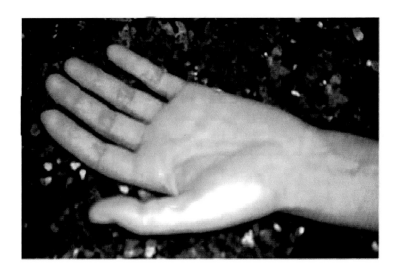

[Fig 9]   Early trophic clawing changes in the hand. (page 35)

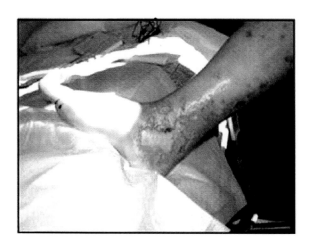

[Fig 10]

Early trophic clawing changes in the hand.
(page 35)

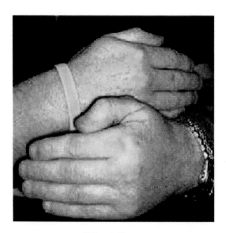

[Fig 11]

CRPS in a hand, but which one? The blue band is a
charity band for RSD UK. The watch is a fake Rolex.
(page 35)

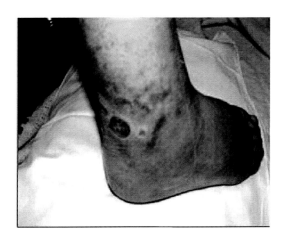

[Fig 12] A severe rash on a CRPS foot (page 35)

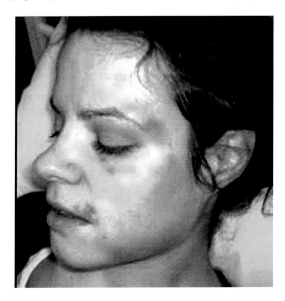

[Fig13] The side of the face of a woman with CRPS of the left hand.
(page 35)
Thanks Naomi, for permission to show these and for the brave smile.

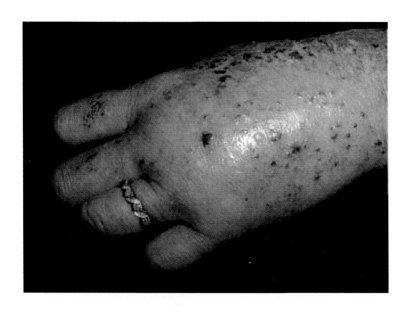

[Figs 14 & 15] Two examples of rashes
(pages 37)

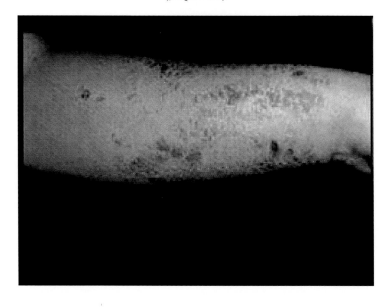

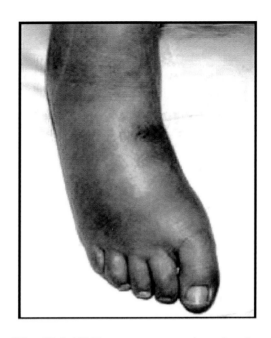

[Figs16 & 17] Two more examples of rashes

(page 35)

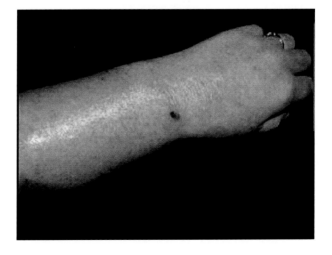

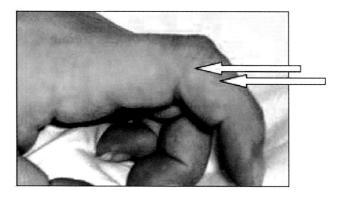

[Fig 18]

Some rashes are much more subtle. Such as this one on the opposite normal hand, it's just a few vesicles that come and go along the edge of the finger. (page 35)

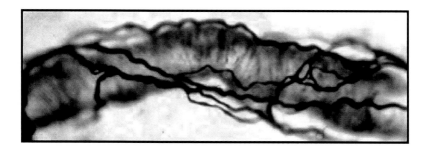

[Fig 19] Fine nerves surrounding very small blood vessels invisible to the naked eye. Large or small nerve damage seems to be the starting point: Image Dr P Mapp (page 38)

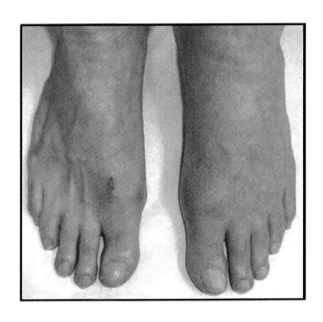

[Fig 20 above] Gout and [Fig 21 below] Infection

Looking a little like CRPS. (page 38)

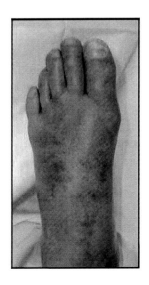

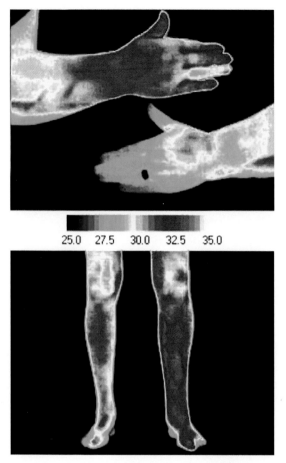

25.0   27.5   30.0   32.5   35.0

[Fig 22 above, Fig 23 below]

Thermograph images showing a CRPS of the left hand and right foot which is colder, but may feel hot. The right hand and left leg are normal. A considerable temperature difference can be felt as a pain as the fine nerves are sensitive to pain. They may feel 'burning' or 'freezing'.(page 40).

Pictures courtesy of Medical Physics, the Neuroscience and Pain Lab. RNHRD, Bath, UK.

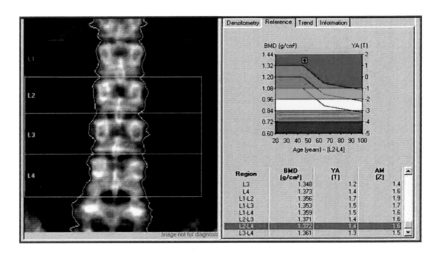

[Fig 24] A Dexa scan and results. (page 47)

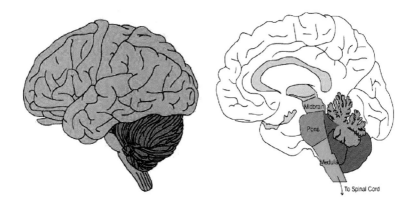

[Figs 25 & 26] The light pink is the cerebrum, the darker the cerebellum and the stem is the brain stem which enlarges into the mid brain. (page 58)

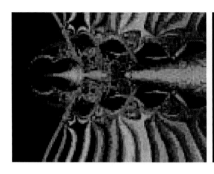 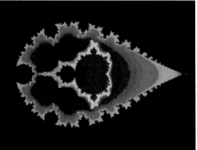

[Figs 27 & 28] These are computer generated fractal pictures and networks may look similar when measured as spikes of electrical activity. Fractals are used especially in computer modelling of irregular patterns and structures in human biology. (page 580)

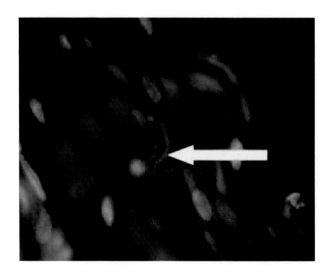

[Fig. 29] Chronic Nerve Compression
Induces Aberrant Axonal Sprouting (page 82)

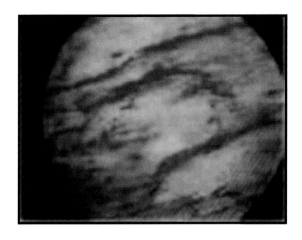

[Fig 30] A bladder wall with Idiopathic Interstitial Cystitis. Swollen blood vessels, oedema and pains.

Is this CRPS? (page 86)

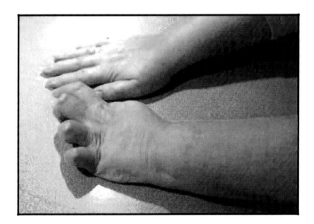

[Fig 31] Locked and clawed for a short time. It occurs after emotional stress or a small bump elsewhere. (page 100)

This was a dog that I had never met before, and the first moment that I met her, like an excited dog she did try and jump up, she did touch my knee, she was told by me and her owner not to do this

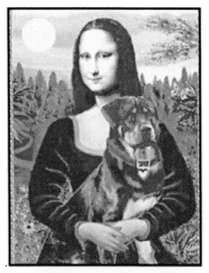 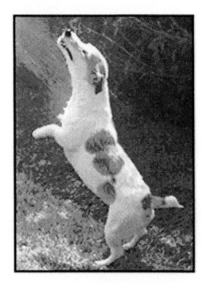

Miss. M. Lisa and Heidi.
From: www.mycraftshowroom.com

Jess

She never came to touch my knee again whilst I was there, but like other dogs she too had a sniff at my knee, but then started to lick the left knee and wasn't happy to stop. I told her to stop, she still continued, but I could feel the licking sensation as if she was licking the right knee. It's hard to explain, I cannot say it hurt, but it felt weird to see a dog licking the left knee for me to feel sensations in my right knee." (This is synchiria, remember?)

Is it possible that these dogs could be detecting a problem with the knee that we cannot smell?"

"… My dogs have learned not to touch my limbs. They do however seem to know when I am having a bad day before the rest do here, they have good senses!"

Here is a "shaggy dog story". This is taken from the Sun newspaper, May 18 2005 so it must be true.

"Dog owner Mitch Bonham had his leg saved from amputation after his pooch LICKED it better."

Mitch had an accident in the Navy leaving him with severe CRPS in his right leg. It was changing colour dramatically, sometimes near black and he and his surgeon anticipated an amputation. Milo the dog, a Jack Russell, did not consider this wise. He licked the limb for up to four hours a day for a year.

When the "consultant saw my leg again he said "my God – what have you been doing? "Incredible, please carry on."

Mitch returned to work with a normal coloured limb.

Mitch says "Milo is one in a million."

Practical problems

Sitting

"I can't explain it. I think the way they explained it to me is that because I've had this condition I lean to the right-hand side which is towards the main injured part.

They say that I do that because of trying to protect it. It's just a natural instinct for me now to do that. But then when they sort of like put me in the correct sitting posture, it just doesn't seem normal to me. In my mind that it feels as if sort of like my head's on my left shoulder. "

Walking and gripping

"Quite a lot of the time, if I'm having a really bad day, I've got to actually look at my right foot to see where it is as I'm walking. It doesn't help when you bump into a lamp post."

"When I was learning to sort of walk again without my sticks I found it incredibly difficult sort of walking from one chair to the other. It's quite bizarre."

"I found it difficult to walk; without crutches I'd lose my balance."

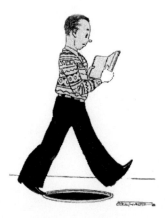

Walking can cause multiple problems.

"The actual sensations on my foot were quite strange because even though I was in considerable pain I didn't have much sensation as far as putting my foot on the floor, I couldn't actually feel if my foot was rested on the floor or what. It seemed to be hanging in mid-air the whole time and that affects my mobility and balance quite a lot."

Using the hand to grip can be very difficult.

"I've got to look at it in order to exercise it. I've got to look at it in order to be able to eat with it. I've got to look at it to be able to pick anything up, to write."

"It's hard to explain but if you want to pick that cup up you only have to look at it once and turn away and your arm would go out and pick that cup up, I couldn't do that. I'd have to concentrate on my hand going to that cup to pick it up. So that's why I'm always looking at it when I exercise".

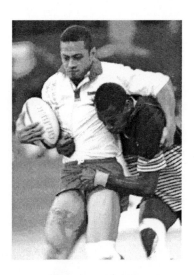

Gripping may be difficult and painful.

"I was told, "Right, move that finger." And I couldn't. If I'd tried to move that finger, the other finger moved. Or if I went to move a finger, two or three fingers would move. So I felt like my hand wasn't attached to my brain. It felt like I really had to concentrate to get that arm going, it was a hard thing to do."

Seeing

"Well sometimes I get like blurred vision."

"Or if I was to turn my head quick you know like the white pixie dust, have you ever seen that?"

"Did I see that? You know, like a box or something, do you know what I mean? I think a little box that moved then."

"For example when I looking round the room at the shelving unit. Well it's as if it flips, the item I look at, it flips, it changes, moves over."

"Well it's like as if, like the DVD case or whatever turns the opposite way."

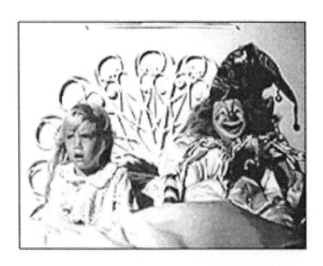

A poltergeist in the house is disturbing.

Most would think they were overrun by a ghost that manifests itself by the creation of disorder: a poltergeist.

Visions

"...not sure what to call these but they aren't much fun. When I wake from sleeping, ten times every night, as soon as I open my eyes I see nothing that should be in my bedroom but like a huge screen of "black flickering snowflakes" - I cant think how else to describe what I see.

They move quite fast towards my eyes; sometimes they are just like black flickering snowflakes but sometimes they take the shape of something else, such as spiders, cats, children, foxes, crabs and these also appear to move towards me, slower than the snowflake ones do.

If I shut my eyes the vision goes, if I open my eyes the vision re-appears.

I had thought, a few years ago they were due to taking amitriptyline but having had several lots of a month or so off them I don't see how it can be as I still got the visions when not taking them."

Reading

"I don't know, wow. See where it's, where you've got the writing starting from the left to the right, you know like ELF yeah? If I stared at that long enough it looks as if it goes over the way, so you've got the E on the opposite side FLE."

"Well I look at people and I think, you know either you've changed or I know you're different, but I can't tell what."

"Sometimes I look at her and I think you look odd today, look strange, but I can't pinpoint what."

"Well I thought, I thought it was my eyes so I went and got my eyes tested, lots of times and my prescription was always changing...odd."

Certainly many, but not all patients with CRPS tell us similar stories. Their world is confusing and simple tasks are difficult.

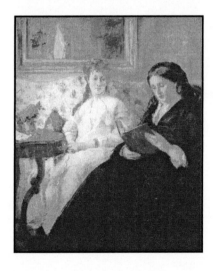

Others may need to read to you or help you with forms.

Artist; Berthe Morisot 1841-1895.

One very important question is the issue of cause and effect. Were there subtle, perhaps hidden perceptual disorders before CRPS developed, or are all these a consequence of the explosive pain reaction firing off closely linked integrated circuits? The answer can of course, be both. A small, barely noticeable, underlying problem may allow for an exaggerated pain response that then magnifies the perceptual problems. This is close to the million dollar question as it allows hypotheses to be developed as to the cause. We could then answer the question "Why me?"

Dreaming

Most of us dream; well all of us it seems, but most can recall the odd dream or two. They are odd for the most part and often the subject of conversation at breakfast. Here's one from the Web:

"I had a dream once that I was in a large white room, sitting at a white table, dressed in white, eating lunch with my boyfriend and two other friends who went out, all three dressed in white. There were no doors or windows on the room, so we were stuck inside. We were just having simple conversations when a gigantic lobster burst through the wall and headed for us. We managed escaping through the hole it made but found ourselves only entering another room just like the one before.

I picked up a long sturdy limb and threw it like a javelin into the lobster's eye, and it shrieked out, died, and shrivelled to the size of a normal lobster. I screamed in my dream, and woke up screaming, in a cold sweat."

Now what's it all about? The dream was unpleasant, irrational and it is hard to see why we all have these dreams. Many of us dream we are flying or running effortlessly which is usually pleasant. Interesting, so do people who have been handicapped for years.

In our rheumatologic practice, a survey of over two hundred patients in the clinic, revealed that over 95% of people with severe arthritis with handicap and in pain were completely normal in their dreams. This is not the case for many CRPS sufferers. Here disability, handicap and importantly pain, travel with you.

Here are some dialogues of dreams.

"When they walked down the beach I could not keep up."

"I dream I have gone to Argos to buy a chain saw to cut off my arm, but when I get home there is no plug."

"And my daughters come into the room with a saw and want to help me and ask if they can cut off my leg. I won't let them."

This seems to be the case in seven out of ten chronic CRPS sufferers. Amputation dreams seem common and distressing.

Dreams are processed in the midbrain and the hippocampus plays a major part. It seems important in creating long and short-term memories allowing rapid associations to be made.

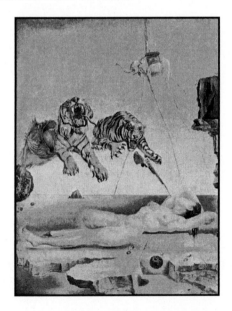

"The difference between false memories and true ones is the same as for jewels: it is always the false ones that look...the most brilliant."

Dreaming. "Index of Sirrobin".
Salvador Dali 1904-1989, a leader of the Surrealist movement.

124

Memories and repetitive thoughts

"My memory is rubbish. I ask the same things over and over again and even important questions or answers can be "lost" in my mind. For example when my son with Aspergers said he was going travelling I was worried about him and I asked him (according to him and the others) no fewer than eight times if he had booked a flight yet. I could not remember asking him or being told the answer. In the end he wrote down his flight numbers etc. If I make a doctors appt I forget, I loose the appointment slip and can't remember if I stored it anywhere and have to ring again to check the time and date three times before I'm happy I know what I am doing. I ask people at work if they have put an order in for me (they have answered, many times, and I can't remember asking them distressing at times - I just want to be how I was."

"Repetitive thoughts are a bloody pain - I must say, before anything else, I have always been told I think too much.

First, it always strikes me odd that I can't remember the things I need to remember without writing it down and setting reminders yet all the stuff floating round my head is trivial rubbish that doesn't need to be stored at all - wish it were the other way round! And this is one of the repetitive thoughts!

Perhaps a lot of my repetitive thoughts though are due to lacking confidence and constantly questioning what I do – but not the necessary things (confusing, sorry).

I keep thinking - how do I know I am doing what I am doing right? Is it because no-one has told me it is wrong? - Most of what I do, I question, then keep thinking about it when I am doing it which is very distracting. E.g. taking an RSD call - the thoughts flick.

"Why is it me they ring?"
"How did I get to here?"
"How do I know I'm doing it right?"

Confusing.

Things like this are very difficult to verbalise because when thinking repetitive thoughts it feels I'm so involved in thinking that I don't

125

remember what they are - and how crazy does that sound! ... And now I'm gonna be thinking about that all the way to work!"

"The other bit - loss of words. Whether typing, writing (which I do little of) or speaking I come to a sudden stop - and that's it.... I can't remember the word, usually one I use daily, really, that is it - but if talking I then can't remember why I needed the word I couldn't remember. If I am typing I write a note in front of me regarding what I was doing, or why I need the word I have lost. Sometimes I never find the right word - it is almost painful trying to find the words, it is a feeling of failure because my memory used to be one thing that I was really proud of.

I feel I spend a good part of each day fumbling round for words, searching everywhere and they just aren't there to recall? It is horrible, truly horrible."

Memory is defined as 'the mental faculty of retaining and recalling past experience.' If we say to you where did you go last for a decent holiday? You may say a holiday in Madeira. Now, we ask, see the hotel lobby and the street to the left. Walk me down it and tell me about the gardens. Off you would go with lots of detail, a cactus, a wild herbal hedge… and around the corner cats asleep…"

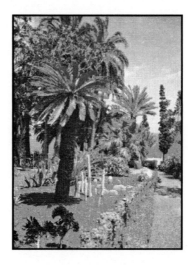

Holidays abroad

126

Now why have you stored that codswallop? What is the point of laying down on your mental hard drive that rubbish? There will be a point otherwise you wouldn't; that's evolutionary biology.

Here is a story: The neurosurgeon, Penfield, who I discussed before, puts a needle into someone's brain in the operating theatre whilst they were conscious.
"What you feel?" he said.
"Nothing" he replied," I can just hear the radio you switched on"
"There is no radio on. What do you hear?"
"Beethoven"
"In what way do you hear it?"
"It's like in a concert."

If I asked you to recall Beethoven's Fifth, presuming you have heard it, you may recall the first few bars. And that's it. What this suggests is that somewhere in your brain is a whole lot more and in glorious technisound. What are these millions, billions of bits of rubbish doing there? Well, they are potentially saving your life. Remember the number of neurones and connections. We have the space on our hard drives to do this.

"I bought a friend a green two-piece; she liked it; I didn't. My mother said green was bad luck, but I told her it was lovely. Now I'm an old man and I'm being mugged and filmed by mindless yobs… what is now called obscenely "happy slappy"… and I am going to die.

I look around, I shout and everyone ignores me… and I see that dress, yes that dress, I shout her name hoping if it is her. She turns, it is, and…" Just a story otherwise I wouldn't be compiling this book. This incidentally is hard work when you are only using two fingers and are dyslexkick.

Those in the know may consider that some of the difficulties with sensory-motor acts have similarities with forms of dyslexia. Indeed imaging and other studies suggest network abnormalities in the temporoparietal language areas.

We create and store all these random bites because one day we may need to access them, link them and do so fast. They are all linked one to another and that's why we think dreams are bizarre; because they are meant to be.

127

Is pain in CRPS such a dominant input that it is subconsciously linked to everything, absolutely everything?

It was said that neonates don't get pain as their cortical brain is immature. This is almost certainly rubbish; remember the lobster with an almost zero cortex and the chef Mr. Ramsey.

Studies of Jewish boys confirmed this to be untrue. Circumcision without any anaesthesia in the first few days of life generates hyperaesthetic (enhanced) responses to different stimuli elsewhere for a considerable time. Is this an example of the deposition of pain in a memory?

We have been doing a few tests of our own on this interesting phenomenon. This is one of them, as a story:

A secretary's tale

"Rachel was my secretary until she moved on to greater things. On this day Rachel is going out to celebrate a friend's birthday and dresses accordingly; meaning high heeled shoes. As all rheumatologists know, these spell trouble in the short and long term.

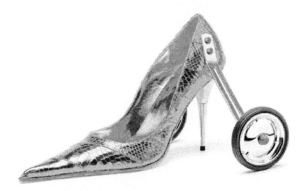

Image from www.basic-consulting.com

The city of Bath has cobbled streets. It is night and Rachel has had two glasses of wine. Her proprioceptive control is chemically impaired, albeit slightly, and darkness impairs and distorts visual clues. The stabilisers get rutted. She falls and twists her ankle badly.

128

She receives attention, has ice and strapping, by a paramedic who loved the shoes, and then had fluctuating pain for twelve days. Since none of the group showed a blind bit of interest she manufactured perceptual outpourings of 'sullen' and did 'body language' which fooled no one.

So we put her in front of a mirror to see if we could make her worse, but told her the opposite.

"Rachel, this is a large mirror and we are putting it between your legs at right angles to you. Now tilt your trunk slightly so you cannot see your injured left one, but you can see your right reflecting in the mirror. Now move each leg out to a comfortable position so that the reflection of your right looks to you as if it's in the position of your left." Here is a picture of Rachel about to have a bad day. We illustrate the procedure with her hand.

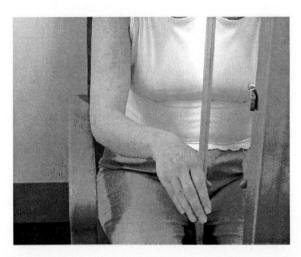

Rachel's brain can 'see' the hidden hand, or is fooled into thinking it can by the mirror.

Now look at me you see I'm moving my ankle up and down. I'm moving my right ankle, the side of your good one as much as I can. Keep the other still. Now look back in the mirror and concentrate only on the reflection for thirty seconds, but only when your left is as pain free as it can be. This she does. Here's a dialogue;

"Now please move the right"

"Ow… you *******"

"What do you feel, describe any pain?"

"My bad ankle is throbbing"

"Where is the throbbing, exactly?"

"Precisely where I twisted it, at the joint edge and below."

"And when did you last feel your ankle that bad?"

"After I sobered up after the party… "

"And when was the last time you had a throbbing pain as opposed to a dull one?"

"Oh, not for weeks."

We think this is important. We could recall the memory of her pain with all its original features without prodding or any movement from the previously injured part. She only moved her healthy ankle. That is a pain from a non-painful stimulus and disproportionate to that stimulus. These are the key initial symptoms and signs of CRPS. Rachel's response however was similar to the pain of the original injury and now presumably a stored memory- fascinating eh?

Can we do this to everyone? No, and the amount we can do it varies considerably between people. We can't get Rachel to experience the same pain now one year later.

"What does it mean said Rachel?"

"You are stark raving mad and should see a shrink…"

But sometime later we told her how it worked and how we had developed the idea. We also told her how we could use the technique to both improve or worsen CRPS without any touch.

We had recently assessed mirror visual feedback (MVF) to test the hypothesis that "incongruence between motor output and sensory input produces complex regional pain syndrome (CRPS type 1) pain".

What does that mean? The explanation is very important as we believe it goes some way to explaining what is going wrong in CRPS. Read this paragraph again and we will explain ourselves. We start by asking, after a brief joke, what incongruence is?

130

A joke is an incongruent input that causes the reflex of laughter. Here is a bad one.

The Bathtub Test

It doesn't hurt to take a hard look at yourself from time to time, and this should help get you started.

During a visit to a mental asylum, a visitor asked the Director what the criterion was which defined whether or not a patient should be institutionalised.

"Well," said the Director, "we fill up a bathtub, then we offer a teaspoon, a teacup and a bucket to the patient and ask him or her to empty the bathtub.

"Oh, I understand," said the visitor. "A normal person would use the bucket because it's bigger than the spoon or the teacup.

"No." said the Director, "A normal person would pull the plug. Do you want a bed near a window?"

Science pain and incongruence

The opposite of incongruence is congruence a term used in lots of disciplines including maths. Here the definition reads "coinciding exactly when superimposed: congruent triangles or squares."

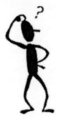 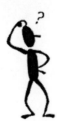

Two congruent men. If you place one on the other you can't see the one underneath.

When Rachel looked at her foot in the mirror we asked her to position it so that it felt that it lay on top of the one she could not see the one obscured behind the mirror. This way she seemed to see the hidden foot. If we had asked her to move her feet together, looking at the reflected image, when the mirror shows her foot to be up, so would the hidden one. Her eyes would be seeing nothing strange. Consequently the feedback from her nerves, that tell her where her foot is, would be congruent with the visual image. We didn't; we asked her to move her foot, but crucially to keep the one that had been injured still. What she saw now was incongruent with what her proprioceptive system was telling her. Her egocentric space was at odds with an allocentric refection. This is a scientific way of saying the same thing.

Proprioception, you recall, is the term we use to describe the very complex mechanisms that tell us where we are in space internally and externally, how we sense ourselves and how we relate to our surroundings. It involves lots of senses, the eyes and the peripheral nervous system and the ears which tell us about which way up we are, and our rotation. Various things happen when you put these in conflict, or to put it another way, engineer their incongruence. Here is an example. Please look at this picture carefully.

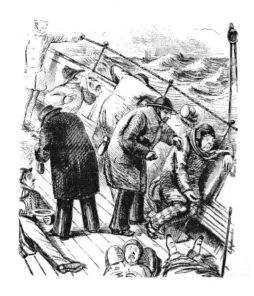

A boat in a storm

We see a boat on rough seas and people with sea sickness. Some seem fine, others are vomiting over the side and some are prostrate.

Motion sickness is a very common disturbance of the inner ear that is caused by repeated variable motion experienced on the sea, in a car, on a plane in turbulent air. In the inner ear (which is also called the vestibular organ or labyrinth), motion sickness affects the sense of balance and equilibrium and, hence, the sense of spatial orientation. It helps to keep the eyes on a fixed point on the horizon if you can. Your proprioceptive system with the visual network is telling you that you are in one place, but the inner ear is feeding a different message or to put it another way, an incongruent signal.

All of us have received the same incongruent stimulus either on a boat or at the fair ground or down the park, but each shows a very different output, from health to illness. Two interconnected reflexes are obvious in motion illness, nausea and vomiting.

If the man leaning over the boat went to his doctor the next day and complained about the motion induced vomiting you would consider the doctor mad if he ordered a barium meal or a gastrosopy to investigate his stomach further. Though the problem manifests itself in the visceral side of the peripheral system, everyone knows, even my mother, that it originates from an incongruent input acting on the brain to cause these peripheral reflexes.

Another incongruent input worth considering as we extend this argument is a rare form of epilepsy. Epilepsy is a brain disorder in which networks of nerve cells in the brain signal abnormally. This causes strange sensations, emotions, and behaviours; sometimes convulsions, muscle spasms, and loss of consciousness.

Photosensitive epilepsy is the name given to a form of epilepsy in which seizures are triggered by flickering or flashing light. Other visual stimuli may do the same. For example, sunlight reflected off wet surfaces or through the leaves of trees, flashing lights in discos and the flickering of faulty fluorescent lighting. Certain geometric shapes or patterns, such as stripes or checks can also do the same.

It is clear that in certain people either auditory or visual inputs trigger specific neuronal networks creating strange and widespread peripheral problems. Dystonia reactions, a regular feature of CRPS, are sometimes preceded by light sensitivity.

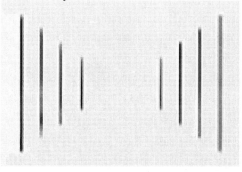

Such images can trigger epilepsy in a minority of epileptics

Could CRPS be a similar process? Perhaps to some extent viewed as an extension of a normal response? We believe the answer is yes.

Migraine also shows some similarities and teaches us a little more. The classical headache, or the rarer warning aura, was considered to be due to blood vessel spasm and widening. Similar views were suggested for CRPS as the blood vessel changes are obvious. The question is what causes this? All blood vessels are surrounded by very fine pain-sensitive nerves as we illustrated earlier. In turn you will recall they contain tiny molecules called neuropeptides. It is now thought that a complex network of electrical activity in the lower brain networks, which comes in waves, triggers activity in select nerves supplying the face and head and send messages to the higher brain, the cortex. The released neuropeptides then act on cells lining our blood vessels, which then release another chemical that causes the blood vessel to react and induces a severe and distressing pain along with characteristic pain behaviours.

The words used to describe the pain are very similar to the words used in CRPS. They have near identical sensory and affective qualities. Neuropeptides will also cause an inflammatory reaction, neurogenic inflammation, which is a complex process involving local oedema and the release of many more chemicals.

The similarities to CRPS pain, vascular changes and inflammation are obvious. The large peripheral nerves involved are clearly different. The fine nerves around the blood vessels will be similar.

What triggers migraine? The answer is lots of things, often quite individual to any sufferer. Hormonal changes, altitude, weather, emotional stress and, you have guessed it, flashing lights and loud sound. These are simple stimuli that are somehow seen as incongruent or treated as if they were and not much different from the stimuli that exacerbate CRPS.

So we start to see links between stimuli that may exacerbate CRPS and also a range of diseases that doctors see as different, but where medical scientists are seeing interesting associations. We have seen similar links when we discussed symptoms such as agnosia in CRPS and compared these symptoms with those generated by specific and apparently different brain disorders. These diseases are sharing overlapping bits of what we are calling the pain network, though we know it does much more than this.

Causing Pain through Incongruent Inputs

We experimented on a number of volunteers to see if an incongruent visual stimulus generated by our mirror technique could cause pain-like perceptions or any other strange, unwelcome symptoms. These are the methods we used and the results. The language should now be understandable to you.

Forty-one, consecutively recruited, healthy adult volunteers, without a history of motor or proprioceptive disorders, performed a series of bilateral upper and lower limb movements whilst viewing a mirror. This created varied degrees of sensory–motor conflict during congruent and incongruent limb movements. A qualitative method recorded any changes in the sensory experience. We used a non- reflective system, a whiteboard, as a control.

Twenty-seven subjects, that is two thirds, reported at least one anomalous or unusual sensory symptom at some stage in the protocol despite no direct peripheral stimulus. The most frequent symptoms occurred when incongruent movement was performed whilst viewing the reflected limb in the mirror condition, the time of maximum sensory–

motor conflict. Symptoms of pain were described as numbness, pins and needles, moderate aching or a definite pain. Other sensations included perceived changes in temperature, limb weight, altered body image and disorientation. There were clear indications that some individuals were more susceptible to generating symptoms than others and some demonstrated pain behaviours. It was not obvious that these were mad, or over excitable, or easily influenced by others, or their surroundings.

So, incongruent visual stimulus generated by a mirror technique can cause pain-like perceptions and other strange, unwelcome symptoms in healthy folk. A proportion gets symptoms, albeit mild, which show some similarity to a CRPS sufferer. Why some and not others is not known, but this could well be genetically based. Some forms of television epilepsy, and epilepsy in general, certainly are as is migraine and dystonia. We do not know, as yet, the genes involved; this however is merely a matter of time and money as the technology available is up to the task, just.

We have a crude idea of where in the brain neuronal activity is stimulated in this experiment. We say crude because the techniques for measuring activity in these networks are imperfect. What we do know from work from Oxford University is that the posterior parietal cortex and the dorsolateral prefrontal cortex on both sides are two of the areas. These areas we have discussed already when we dissected neglect and agnosia.

Relieving Pain through Congruent Inputs

Professor Vilayanur Ramachandran, a medical doctor, is Director of the Centre for Brain and Cognition and Professor within the Psychology Department and the Neurosciences Program at the University of California, San Diego. He wrote, with Sandra Blakeslee, a New York Times Science writer, the critically acclaimed book 'Phantoms in the Brain.' This is a must for further reading it is clear,   easy to follow, and deals with problems similar to ours.

Using mirrors he was the first to alleviate a pain state. The condition which interested him was amputation or phantom pain. They asked people with amputations of the arm and subsequent phantom limb pain to place their arms inside a mirror box. They saw their remaining arm mirror-reversed to look like their amputated one in the same way we have described. When they moved their arm in the box the brain was 'fooled' into thinking they were moving their amputated one. Their pain was reduced. The results were not uniform, some responded very well, others much less; in a few it was dramatic. Prof V Ramachandran however had a problem. How do you measure pain in a limb that is not there? You could of course image the brain and we have seen a picture, but how do you know that is pain and not the emotional response to it. Perhaps it does not matter.

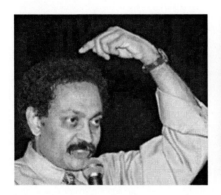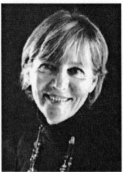

Vilayanur S. Ramachandran MD, PhD. and Sandra Blakeslee

Photo Joan Myers, William Morrow Joan

Now let us return to CRPS; recall our hypothesis, "We had assessed mirror visual feedback to test the hypothesis that 'incongruence' between motor output and sensory input produces complex regional pain syndrome pain." It will be clear now why we did this.   Incongruent feedback via a mirror stimulates the cortex. In some normal volunteers it can cause pain. In Rachel it restored a pain memory. We did the same experiment on a volunteer with CRPS and her pain was worsened. Now we are ready to test the opposite state. Our hypothesis is that "creating congruence, by visual imagery, between motor output and sensory input reduces Complex Regional Pain Syndrome." These were our results.

Eight subjects were studied over six weeks and asked to use a mirror box-like system and make small and ever-increasing congruent movements. In the hands, for example, we would ask patients to open and close the fingers as much as possible; both hands doing exactly the same movement, otherwise it is incongruent movement. The diseased hand was hidden and vision confined to the reflected site of the normal hand superimposed on the painful one by the mirror arrangement. We measured pain severity using a scale we describe later. The temperature of the limb was measured by thermography. In patients with early disease and without trophic changes the results were dramatic. Pain relief came within a minute and with increasing exposure to the mirror lasted for longer and longer, creating effective cures in some in a few weeks. In longer-lasting disease the results were more variable. The temperature changes resolved as did the swelling/oedema, phantom or true.

Subsequent studies by us and others have confirmed this exciting finding and we have learnt, both with and through others, how to improve the response.

We now turn to treatment programmes and the key message here is 'one size does not fit all', chill and be patient.

Before you get into a specialist programme for CRPS pain management you will need to see a medical consultant for review. The following is what you might expect.

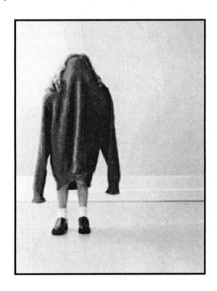

'One size does not fit all', but since kids wear fashionable clothes that don't fit anyway - who cares? From www.okea.org

Treatment and beyond

Visiting a hospital consultant

Doctors come in all shapes and sizes and their personalities do the same. You can reasonably expect courtesy and a professional informed opinion, but don't bank on liking us. That would be a bonus. If I was seeking my perfect doctor he would conform to this model.

> Give me a doctor partridge plump,
> Short in the leg and broad in the rump,
> An endomorph with gentle hands
> Who will never make absurd demands
> That I abandon all my vices
> Nor pull a long face in a crisis,
> But with a twinkle in his eye
> Will tell me that I have to die.
>
> W. H Auden (1907-1973)
> British poet.

Unfortunately we know of no such doctor.

Let us start with a few words about a clinic and what to expect; a few do's and don'ts. It is very unlikely, if you are reading this with an established diagnosis, that the following is not obvious. However patients behave like tourists in airports and if there is a clearly wrong way they leap at it. They all do, observe them.

A hospital clinic is different from your family doctor's surgery and it is an alien environment for many. It is intimidating to some. We write from the perspective of the UK NHS and are aware that different health systems operate in other ways. One of us conducted a clinic abroad with nursing

139

support and no less than twenty patients in the examination hall at once. Relatives, friends and one goat all attended.

A few simple rules

- Come with time to settle.
- Don't be angry if the doctor is delayed.
- Smile even if it's an effort.
- Be courteous and expect courtesy in return.
- Expect to be hurried. A 'new patient' appointment is thirty minutes, a 'follow up' fifteen. [Why? You may well ask!]
- Turn off your mobile phone and please avoid bringing food, drink or chewing gum into the clinic.

Expect to have 'a history' taken, both specific to your problem and more general. The doctor will require a full list of drugs you are on, often the drugs you have taken previously and any allergies or unwanted effects that you have experienced. Write these down in capitals with the drug dose and time taken. State clearly, and in writing, if they worked or not. Be honest about whether you take them. Tell the doctor if you have been prescribed drugs, but not taken them for some reason (many don't). Write down any complimentary medicines you have received and any benefits or problems.

Expect to be examined thoroughly. Wear underwear you are not embarrassed to show others. Expect to be asked to remove socks and tights for this.
An examination of a patient with a rheumatic disease usually involves a full examination of the 'locomotor system' including gait, balance, arms, legs and spine. We need to see it. Examining a CRPS patient involves more. If embarrassed or nervous or plain scared, bring a relative or friend as an escort. It is rare to find a nurse assistant in an examination room. In clinics with a lot of experience of CRPS they will respect your wish not to prod or poke the painful part. If not, explain your difficulties without anger. In our clinics we do the CRPS bit last or after you have a break.

This is what is involved and presumes a common site for CRPS such as the hand or leg.

140

We have discussed all the key features already. Pain is the most important, but we get to that last.

First we look. Is it swollen, and how far does the swelling extend? Is the swelling uniformly distributed? What is the colour and is it uniform or mottled? Are the nails distorted? Is there abnormal hair growth? Is there abnormal sweating? What is the position of the limb, foot or hand? Are there abnormal dystonic movements or postures? Can you make a grip or curl you foot? If asked to reach for an object how do you do it? If we ask you to move, say a finger, is that what moves? We do not touch you.

Then we get you to test for pain examining light touch, a blunt pinprick and temperature. Then we assess if your touch feels the same as a stranger's touch. We have all the information from the questionnaire, but now we add detail. We assess what movements you can do without pain and what you can't. If the answer is very few we examine you for just the consequence of imagined movements. All the time we look at the colour and the sweating. We monitor your anger, frustration and hostility threshold. We observe you for depressive type signs or passive aggression. At the end we have a good idea of the extent of your allodynia under stressful conditions. A clinic is a stress. It usually heightens pain perceptions and adverse secondary perceptual difficulties become obvious.

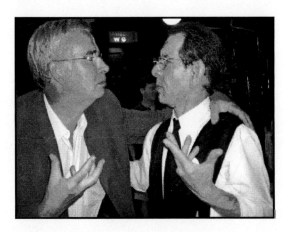

A spot of anger and stress between an author and a French waiter.
Occasionally anger is justified. The soup was cold.

Expect to be sent for investigations to assess the CRPS and exclude diseases that may look similar. We have discussed many of these already. You may be reassessed again after these initial tests. In multidisciplinary clinics, such as ours, the total time may be quite considerable. At this point, if time permits or at another session, we observe and examine for perceptual problems.

You will then receive an explanation of what is found and be provided with information to read and discuss with others. This book might be on offer in which case this advice is clearly too late.

You may well be present when the doctor dictates a report to the referring doctor; this is to allow you to correct any mistakes. If you need a report for your employer or legal advisor this is the time to ask.

Keep smiling from time to time.

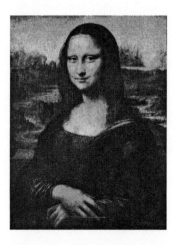

A smile with composure

Ask questions; usually best at the end. If you forget those that are important to you write them down, ready for next time. If you bring a relative try not to let them answer on your behalf. Your words matter. If you say the pain is agonising we believe you; if a colleague answers for you it can mean anything.

142

Ask any colleague to listen carefully and then chat about it later to help your memory. Try, if possible, not to let them scribble notes. Remember you will receive a report.

> If you sight a chief executive or senior health manager please remember to bow or curtsy. The same rule applies for middle, lower- middle, upper- lower, lower, lower- lower, acting-up, acting-down and trainee grade managers.
> The repeated exercise is helpful which leads us to...

Now prepare treatment plans. These are individualised to your needs- where we are permitted. The programme is extensive, and extensive means time, and time means money. Rehabilitating CRPS is effective, but expensive. Resources within our National Health Service are limited, financially rationed and prioritised. Pain and rheumatological services are not priorities and resources are overstretched. This is a political issue. It is our responsibility to lobby on behalf of our patients' needs. It is also yours to lobby on behalf of yours, others and ours. Lobbying usually is successful if it is vocal repetitive and verging on extreme. It would certainly help if someone famous or notorious had this condition and was prepared to speak up. Anyone fit?

The proportion of patients on the RSD/CRPS database who responded with help to support this book with stories and experiences was low. However, the proportion who complained of difficulties accessing services, often established voluntarily, is high. The high complaint rate of chronic pain suffers against the medical professions makes many reluctant to join this sub-specialty and develop the service.

How to get things better as quickly as possible

Physiotherapy is the only proven therapy for CRPS. This specialist service uses physical agents such as exercise and massage and other modalities to help.
Sufferers' reactions to physiotherapy are extreme, from radiant to appalling. Physiotherapy can help nearly everyone, but the key to success is a good assessment, an individually tailored programme and time. Patience, determination, doggedness and resolve are the key to success.

A full assessment is time-consuming, difficult and often outwith the experience of a general physiotherapist. What are the questions you should ask yourself prior to physiotherapy and should be asked of you? Here are ours. They relate to pain and the linked perceptual problems we have discussed.

We have written this in the form of a postal questionnaire we are presently assessing. We are not asking you to do it and send it to us. We present it so you can see where we are coming from. However you may wish to have a go as it helps to reinforce the text. The assessors will be patients, doctors and allied health professionals. The questionnaire is based on an analysis of patients' response from the RSD annual conference 2005. The attendees had both CRPS type 1 and 2. They predominately had protracted disease; both children and adults participated, many accompanied by their carers. Details of the programme are available from the RSD UK Web address listed under 'essential reading' at the end.

It will be modified over time and is being personalized appropriately for face to face assessments. The questions are essentially the same, but the style and approach customised for the spectrum of ages seen in the clinic. Whilst it is time saving and useful to have information prior to reviews, there are drawbacks. In particular, patients with CRPS have difficulty concentrating and indeed written text that is crowded may occasionally be blurred and shimmer and ddo (odd).

Questionnaire

PLEASE READ THE ENTIRE QUESTIONNAIRE FULLY BEFORE YOU COMPLETE IT.

Example only

It is in sections A-I. Please follow the instructions carefully.

You may prefer to complete the form with a carer or friend. Please ask him/her to say nothing when you respond. It is your answers we need.

Section A

Is English your first language?   If the answer is no, please do not proceed. We will complete this with you in the clinic and perhaps you can help us with a translation.

Do you have more than one separate site of pain? For example Right arm/left leg/face.

Where is your **worst** pain (just one site)?

Do you have different kinds of pain?   Please list all of them here. Examples may be burning, shooting and throbbing. There are lots more. What are yours? Give up to 10.

1	6
2	7
3	8
4	9
5	10

Which of these pains is the one you find the worst at this moment?
For example the 'throbbing' or the 'gnawing'.

If 10 is the worst you have ever experienced this pain and 0 is no pain where would you put your present pain on the line below? Mark the line.

0 _____10

Where is your second worse pain?

0 _____10

Please mark the line using the same scale.

If I had asked these questions two days ago would they have been the same?

If not, how would they be different?

Section B

Please take a break before completing the rest of the form.

If these questions are not relevant please mark NR. Please do not leave any space or box blank. The answers decide which of our physio programmes is best for you. We have eight different programmes.

You are sitting in a chair, your worst part is exposed and a stranger walks slowly toward you. Would you have any worsening of the pain? (If 'no' then please takes no notice of the next four questions.) Please try it for real, if there is an 'on hand' ... stranger. If this important pain test is positive let it settle before proceeding.

If positive, guess/ record how close they could come up to you. Is it within an inch, a foot, a yard or further? Is it five, ten, centimetres or a metre? Remember we are talking of pain only.

If yes, did you feel 'panicky'?

Section C

Please take another rest. The next appraisal is a practical one and must be done with someone you trust.

Please expose your worst affected area. Ask your chosen friend to sit beside you at least a yard/metre away and move his or her hand towards you.

Could he/she touch you before you felt pain?

146

Please touch your worst part, or as nearby as you can tolerate. Press just hard enough to make it hurt a little.

Describe the pain. Now let it clear up.

Please take your friend's hand and touch yourself with it .The same heaviness should be applied and for the same length of time.

Now describe the sensation noticing any difference from your earlier response. Now let it clear up.

Section D

Do you have swelling of the worst part?

Can you see it?

Can your friend see it?

Does it feel the same with your eyes shut? Close your eyes for a minute and try it.

Is the swelling you feel different from the swelling you see and how?

If it is different is it in exactly the same place?

Section E

Is your worst part stiff and for how long each day?

What time of day are your symptoms generally worse.
Presuming you don't work night-shifts is it morning, afternoon evening or in bed?

Does the pain wake you at night?

Is the pain any different at night?

Can you cope with bed clothes touching you?

Is there any item of your clothing you don't like to wear? For example shoes, gloves or socks perhaps?

Section F

Does your bladder feel full when it should not?

How soon after going to the toilet does it start to feel over full.

Do you have trouble with pain around your backside (anus?)
Do you experience pain on or in your penis or vagina?
If your hand/ foot are affected and you touch it hard do you feel pain in your face or around your bottom?

PLEASE TRY IT.

Does it work the other way round? Face (scratch) and then a hand feeling: Bottom (scratch) and then a foot feeling?

Section G

Now for some rather strange questions; they are not trick questions or put in to see if you are a little crazy. They are feelings many people with certain forms of RSD/CRPS get.

Does your arm or foot feel like it belongs to you?

Does your arm or foot have missing bits?

Is it always in the place that you can see, or do you sometimes feel it has moved when it has not?

Does your hand or foot have a life of its own and move when you do not want it to?

Does it always move correctly where you expect? For example if you try to move one finger, is this always the one that moves?

Do you sleep well?

Finally, in your dreams are you disabled at all, or is everything normal?

Section H

When you look at faces of people do they seem blurred?

If you look at familiar things in the room do they move when they should not?

Do flickering things cause you difficulties? For example lights or objects seen from a moving car or train?

Before you had CRPS was everything normal or did you have any difficulties with how you saw external objects?

Before CRPS did you ever feel really bloated anywhere?

Section I (and the end.)

Put your affected (bit) hand or leg in a comfortable position.
Now with your eyes closed imagine you are moving it for a minute. What did you feel?   Thank you

Interpreting the questionnaire and planning treatments

From this simple information, which is coupled to a detailed history and examination, we can start to move forward. We describe a programme based on a worst case situation.

That would be a patient with allodynia to threat only and with poor perceptual control of the limb and dystonic reactions. For this illustration we assume the CRPS is in the upper arm between hand and elbow.

We assume 'neglect-like' features coupled with a sense that the limb is alien and that there is evidence of referred sensations to the face on testing. Such a patient would make a poor response to immediate traditional physiotherapy and may well be worsened by it.

Desensitising allodynic pain to touch

On the basis of our present knowledge, which is imperfect, the first stage to progress would be to explain that all parties must commit to the long haul.

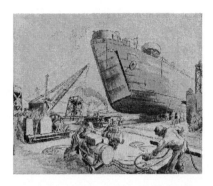

The Long Haul - Thomas Hart Benton

Then we reduce the perceived threat of touch. This is best done by the sufferer in the first instance. We have heard already of the man who got his dog to lick him better. This is what he was doing, desensitising himself, and then the colour changes occurred. Remember the dog worked on him for four hours a day for a year.

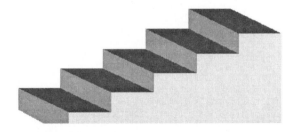

Desensitisation is a slow and gentle process…

You start by touching yourself with any thing you find not painful, or minimally so, and you repeat and repeat and repeat. When you have finished you repeat the process again and again until it's a reflex.

150

When going to sleep think touch exercises, making breakfast think touch exercises and, after a while, build the intensity of the stimulus, do it a little firmer and later do it with a more textured stimulus. Then ask someone you like and trust to do it for you.

Take the stimuli with you when you go out and carry on doing it: in cars, trains, on the bus and in the cinema indeed, anywhere where two things can be done at once. Occupational therapists can teach you if you have difficulties, though the most common difficulty is not doing it.

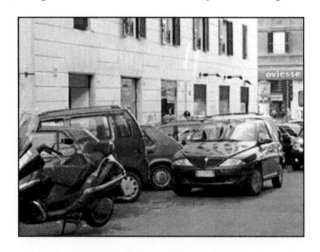

"Rome was not built in a day"
"but Italians may wonder" as they still screwed up the parking system.
[Anagram]

Imagine making a grip

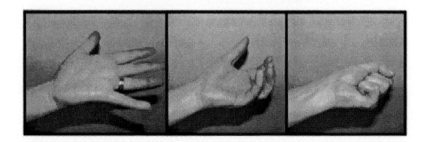

The first step is to do no more than imagine you are doing this in small stages. You practice with your good hand first until you have the knack, looking at the pictures initially and then without. 'Rome rule' applies and this takes time to master, but soon you can do it anywhere, and all the time.

Making a simple grip

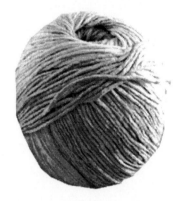

Cotton or wool made into a ball.

This can be adjusted in size to make it easy to grip.

The patient does no more than play with it, rolling between the good and bad hand for ages. When the pain sensation is reduced to a minimal level you should extend the rubbing further up the arm. Look at the limb constantly and then without observation. It's a good idea to put yourself in any environment you find relaxing. Listening to soft music suits many.

This step is boring but essential and should only be abandoned in favour of stage two when the stimulus is nearly inert. Then start making a grip reducing the size of the ball as you progress. Do it everywhere. Then change the gripped object to a tube or a box, whatever takes you're fancy as long as it gets a little more difficult. You can link this with the exercise below as you progress.

Doing small movements repeatedly

Make the smallest movement that causes no pain. Again always choose the same relaxing environment. Please look at the hand when doing the exercise, then brief periods looking away.

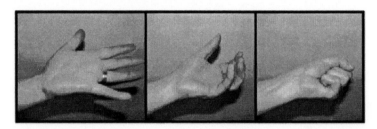

Never ever rush.

In this programme pain lessens gain considerably. There is no set period for these three simple stages. Try to think in terms of weeks though this varies enormously.

Using a mirror

Buy or borrow a large mirror and set it up at right angles from you in a comfortable chair and environment. Get someone to secure it firmly at the base. Try to make it a permanent (-ish), so that you can do the exercises a lot. Most people with all these programmes, try once, say it is hopeless and abandon ship. Not a good idea.

Remember the dog.

Ours is secured on a purpose-built frame that allows it to be adjusted for different people. We angle it so the reflected image is perfectly superimposed on the injured part, either the hand or foot. Do no more, to start with, than practice viewing the image in the glass and creating the illusion it is your injured hand. Again spend loads of time on this and don't proceed until you are both relaxed and comfortable with the illusion. Holding a limb up in the mirror may create pain: position the limbs or support them until this is nil. Here are a few dialogues from patients with longstanding CRPS.

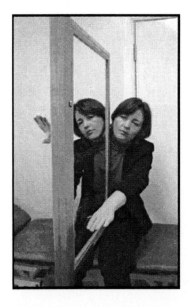

Left: Using a mirror repeatedly for graded rehabilitation; put a large one on a door. Perhaps a flexible mirror; light and easy to pivot and remove. (Model Jenny Lewis)

"They said, you know, 'Maybe you'd like to try this'. Basically you had to look in a mirror and, for a while, get my eyes used to that. Then I had to look in the mirror with my left hand, get my right hand on the other side so I couldn't see my right hand and then see if by moving my left hand my right hand would move. Actually, believe it or not, as stupid as it sounds, it worked. And it was a brilliant way of exercising in the beginning, and it's still a very good way of exercising now. I do it loads."

"I've been having a go at mirror therapy as well which again has been quite brilliant when I've actually been doing the mirror because, although you know you're kidding your brain, some how it works and I don't pretend to understand how it works. But the first time for a very, very long time my arm, my right arm has looked like it has been behaving normally."

"That has helped a lot with the pain and immediately after the mirror my arm feels an awful lot better."

"I think at this stage yeah I've been told that it's a long haul and I'm looking at a year plus, it'll be very slow steps so you can't hope for miracles overnight."

"I'm aiming for at least eight times a day for five minutes each session.

154

> Which is right; little and often.

Desensitising yourself to other allodynic stimuli other than touch by counter conditioning

People differ here. There are so many stimuli; lights flashing, noise, colours on white backgrounds. The list is endless. The principles of desensitisation are similar for all. These pain-inducing stimuli are all associated with anxiety at some level and both anxiety and pain can be deconditioned by what we call reverse 'Pavlovian therapy'.

Ivan Pavlov was born in a small village in central Russia eventually becoming the professor of Physiology at the Imperial Medical Academy.

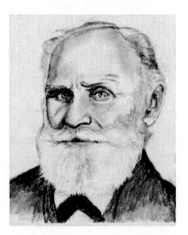

Ivan Pavlov (1849-1936)

The work that made Pavlov famous throughout the scientific world began as a study in digestion.

He was looking at the process in dogs, especially the interaction between salivation and the action of the stomach. He realized they were closely linked by reflexes in the autonomic nervous system and parallels are obvious with allodynia and colour changes in CRPS.

Without salivation, the stomach didn't get the signal to digest food.
Pavlov wanted to see if an external stimulus could affect this process. He rang a metronome at the same time he gave the experimental dogs food. After a while, the dogs would begin to salivate when the metronome sounded, even if no food were present. In 1903 Pavlov published his results calling this a 'conditioned reflex', different from an innate reflex, such as yanking a hand back from a flame, in that it had to be learned. Pavlov called this learning process 'conditioning'. He also found that the conditioned reflex will be subdued and eventually stop if the stimulus proves 'wrong' too often. If the metronome sounds repeatedly and no food appears, the dog will after a while stop salivating at the sound. This is why we call it reverse Pavlovian therapy.

The trick is to associate a small amount of the signal with relaxation in some form. The relaxation you choose for yourself and then you slowly introduce the stimulus in ever increasing amounts. A carer comes in very useful as he or she can deliver the stimulus. Again the technique works, but it takes time and patience.

Hands on physiotherapy and occupational therapy

Once intervention from a partial stranger does not induce an allodynic response, traditional physiotherapy with manipulation, exercises and desensitisation will work in most and particularly early in the disease. It takes longer if CRPS is well established. Varieties of modalities are used to encourage movement. Passive and active movements are the mainstay of the programme; both can be done at home.

Your physiotherapist will show you and your carer which passive exercise would be most of use.
Active movements are the same, but without help from another.

156

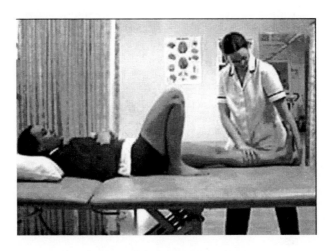

From www.mndcentre.org.uk

How successful they are depends on how extreme the allodynic pain response is and how labile the symptoms are.

Acupuncture, electrotherapy and trans-cutaneous nerve stimulation can help individuals if the allodynia is minimal. Many, however, report considerable problems if acupuncture is started too early.

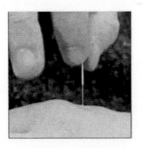

Acupuncture
thejadetrade.net

Trophic changes can be serially splinted to limit deformities, but they often pop back to the previous position as the problem is rarely a fixed contracture. Legs and arms will reposition themselves when the CNS is desensitised, and not before. Too rigorous splinting can make things worse as it creates a Pavlovian conditioned reflex.

Difficulties with every day tasks such as dressing, fastening buttons or zips, preparing or eating a meal and managing tasks such as writing, holding a book, opening a purse, can all be helped by a skilled occupational therapist.

Assistance can now be obtained from alternative health providers. Specialists in Yoga and Pilates help with overall suppleness.

Yoga

"There are several forms and paths of yoga that include meditation (Raja Yoga), devotional prayer (Bhakti Yoga), selfless service to others (Karma Yoga), practices for discrimination of truth and reality (Jnana Yoga), and even meditational forms of exercise and bodily upkeep (Hatha yoga, a part of Raja Yoga)."

From www.explainplease

Pilates

The core fundamentals of the Method are based upon a thorough understanding of the anatomy of the human body. The Pilates Teacher uses this information to create a comprehensive exercise programme for each client with the aim of restoring a greater sense of balance. It is this holistic approach that sets the Method apart from many other forms of exercise.
www.pilatesfoundation.com

Relaxation, hypnosis and self control

We have seen much evidence for the profound effects psychological factors play in pain perception; many positive, some negative, some profoundly so. What's to be done?

To tackle this very important question, and for a bit of fun, we discuss what psychology is. Here are three definitions from the web:

Philosophy: the branch of metaphysics that studies the soul, the mind, and the relationship of life and mind to the functions of the body.
Scientific: the science that deals with mental processes and behaviours.

Lay perception: the emotional and behavioural characteristics of an individual.

Dealing with the philosophical, we are invited to understand what is metaphysics and soul. We looked this up for you and here it is; "The branch of philosophy that examines the nature of reality. This includes the relationships between mind and matter, substance and attribute, fact and value." Help!

It gets better when we come to soul. "The animating and vital principle in humans credited with the faculties of thought, action, and emotion and often conceived as an immaterial entity."

Many would debate the existence of an immaterial entity. Whilst we know relatively little about the networks relating to kindness, hatred, anger and joy we know enough to understand that the system works like the pain network with which it connects. Namely it's a series of complex electrical discharges, driven by chemical reactions, under genetic control and modifiable by experience based on memories. The latter is also a brain network. These networks are clearly not "immaterial".

The issues are scientific and relate to understanding how to control our psychological reactions.

For those who are religious, of any faith, calling upon memories generated by knowledge and based on a belief system may be a start. Some might say that faith influences on health are little more than positively conditioned Pavlovian reflexes. For those who are not religious there is plenty to be done to gain control with help or on ones' own.

The lay definition is fine.
It is vital to remember we have some control and being passive is not sensible; indeed it is harmful. This section is a rough guide to making

progress. Rough, as none of the authors has had a training in psychology, so there is plenty of scope for you to disagree with us.

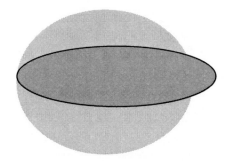

Pain is dark, psychology is light. Pain and psychology co-exist or to put it another way, there is no pain without attention.

The two intimately coexist, with the possible exception of acute unexpected reflex pain which may escape for a second or two.

Pain occurs, associated with varying degrees of distress, unless it is related to sexual pleasure - the latter being a minority taste.

In CRPS with allodynia, distress is a universal accompaniment of the pain experience. Helplessness, or the feeling of helplessness, is a critical factor and relates directly to the intensity of pain. Depression or anger may be a consequence of the sense of helplessness as we have seen. Learning control, through relaxation, is a key element of treatment and indeed is fundamental to the physiotherapy and occupational therapy programmes described.

Let us start by considering enhanced relaxation and hypnosis. Historically, hypnosis was defined as 'an altered state of consciousness, characterized by heightened compliance with suggestion and extreme focused attention.'

Hypnosis has been used as a pain management tool with considerable success in some disciplines, particularly dentistry. MRI studies to image the brain and define which networks are influenced have been applied to study the scientific effects.

160

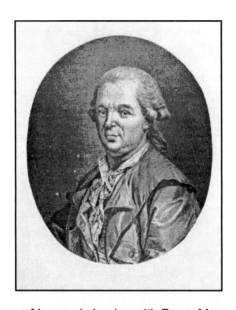

The recent history of hypnosis begins with Franz Mesmer (1734-1815), who theorized that disease was caused by imbalances of a physical force, called animal magnetism. In 1784, a French royal commission chaired by Benjamin Franklin concluded that the effects of mesmerism, while genuine in many cases, were achieved by means of imagination and not by any physical force. Mesmer's theory was discredited.

Hypnosis is not about loss of control. Successful hypnosis is concerned with creating a state of extremely focussed attention which allows you to move away from damaging attentive drivers. It is similar to reading a riveting book or watching an intensely captivating film. Here you can be so consumed with the stimulus that you are oblivious to all others. In such a state pain is modified.

If another person is hypnotising you, his suggestions in this focussed state can increase or decrease pain. This we have done in our own laboratory and we found it is possible to recall a previous pain from memory and respond to it as if it were a fresh stimulus; the response is accompanied by all the same secondary reflex characteristics of distress, sweating, fast pulse and faster breathing. The opposite is also the case. Part of the control of CRPS involves learning such techniques and applying them into your total physiotherapy package.

Chronic allodynic pains are worse when you return from work in the evening due to the lack of distractions. It is not due to being a little tired.

There are a variety of techniques exploited by hypnotists and those who self hypnotise. Much depends on your susceptibility to hypnotism which is assessed by a trained hypnotist who utilises the Stanford Hypnotic Susceptibility Scale. There are 12 standard tests in the susceptibility scale which measure how well a subject conforms to the behaviour of a classically hypnotised person. By these scales, about 5% of people are classically un-hypnotisable, most people show moderate scores, and about 10% are hypnotizable to extreme depths and show deep trance phenomena such as sleep walking, visual and auditory hallucinations, and ability to remain hypnotised with their eyes open.

Hypnotisability does not appear to show any obvious correlation with any of the usual personality traits or characteristics. Gullibility is not directly correlated, neither are gender, extraversion-introversion, and neurotic tendencies.

Hypnosis involves the use of images and metaphors/similes. These serve to help filter the hurt or suffering component out of the pain perception. The pain is acknowledged or accepted but the person is trained to distinguish between the sensation in and the perception out. This we discussed in detail at the start of this little book. Pain is then transformed as a perception into something less disagreeable like warmth or coolness or numbness. You are trained not to fight the pain which only creates more attention to it. You are trained to relax sufficiently to transform the pain. Combinations of imagery and relaxation are used. Again much of this is positive Pavlovian conditioning.

To assist in self-hypnosis, you need to master what are known as induction techniques. Using these many can self-hypnotise within seconds. It works most effectively if you put specific and regular parts of the day aside so that routines are established. Self-hypnosis is not the same as having a brief nap, you must stay awake. Many find it best to practice lying down, in a comfortable position, with as few distractions as possible.

Hypnotic induction is divided into four stages, relaxation, deepening, suggestion, application and termination. Relaxation is to get you physically relaxed, your mind then follows. This is not so easy with

162

CRPS, but it is achievable with patience. Every part of the body needs to become limp and relaxed.

Whilst initially the CRPS limb will not do so, with time it will follow to increasing degrees. Tensing each of the major muscle groups of your body in a strict pattern helps, but ignores the CRPS limb. To deepen the states of relaxation count down from two hundred at a natural speed in time with your breathing. Breathing rates will slow down, so counting slows.

Relaxation and deepening needs to be practiced for a good length of time before the next stage is developed. This may be months for some. Relaxation alone alters the network. Relaxation is not the same as not attending. You are initially attending to relaxation until lower brain activities take over and do it reflexly for you. That is why your breathing slows as autonomic activity is driven less by the sympathetic nervous system and more by the parasympathetic. These 'fright and flight' and 'chill out responses' we have discussed and illustrated.

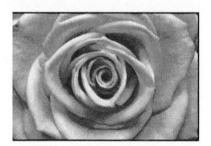 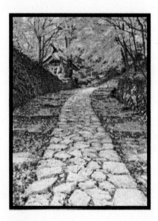

Hypnotic images may help
in the deepening phase.

Work out the suggestions for the next phase of deepening well in advance and mesmerise them both as words and images. [Now you know where the word mesmerise comes from, yes Franz Mesmer.] They need to be short and simple images that help you relax. Many find recalling aspects of a stress free day on holiday works. For example think yourself walking slowly through a park. Once deepened, or partially so, introduce exercises in your mind very slowly. Imagine the ball of wool and your fingers gently squeezing it in a pain free fashion. You don't make it more difficult until this is achieved, eventually taking a real ball of wool with you when you do the exercises. Later consider the limb slightly numb and slowly develop the feeling so exercise and numbness associate in the memory. This is now changing part of the pain network.

You should identify the end of every session quite distinctly. This helps to demarcate between the hypnotic state and your ordinary state. It also helps to stop you going off to sleep.

Hypnotic analgesia exercises change electrical activity in the brain as measured by a technique known to scientists as "event-related brain potentials". The electrical activity is reduced to potentially painful stimuli. Other techniques have established changes where and suggest this may happen in an area of the brain known as the anterior cingulate gyrus. The anterior cingulate gyrus is the part of the brain that registers conscious emotion. It communicates between the prefrontal cortex and sub cortical areas of the limbic system including the hippocampus and amygdala. The hippocampus we discussed when we talked about perceptual problems with cubes and other stimuli. The amygdala is concerned with our fears. It rapidly stimulates the autonomic system, generating the sympathetic fright and flight response.

Enhanced relaxation inducing analgesia is certainly no game or placebo. Given our relative lack of drugs, we consider hypnosis or enhanced relaxation a useful player for many in a treatment programme. Here are some dialogues.

"…about four or five sessions with him. He put me under the very first session and he said I was easy to put under, I knew he was doing it. I wasn't a case that he could turn round and say "Right, take your shoes off and pretend you're a chicken" because I would just turn around and say 'get stuffed'. It wasn't that types of 'under' you see on television. But he did say, like your arms are totally light- weight there's no weight in it whatsoever, it's just going to float up and …there is my arm floating up.

He said I was a very easy subject and "Well, I ought to just try and teach you how to do it for yourself".

"It helped and it would last maybe a day, two days. Total, total relief, no pain whatsoever just a numb hand and arm."

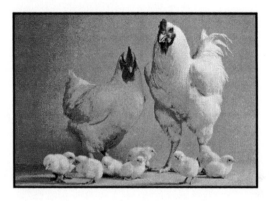

From www.cvm.msstate.edu/ Poultry/Images

"One thing I have tried, and it's really helped, and that's hypnotherapy. It's been fantastic and I think that helped me in actually getting my limb to move and helped with pain because, a hypno-therapist I used, he's very good and he does this thing, I can't remember what it's called now but it's 'tapping' and it works. I don't know how it works, but it works."

"I would recommend hypnotherapy because it is connected, you know, the brain has a massive part to play in this condition, well the main part probably of this condition, so I'd definitely say to anybody give this a go."

Not everyone can truly relax: here is a story sent by someone who found their symptoms worsen when they tried.

"How do I feel nine years or so on with CRPS?"

"Things could be worse, I tell myself, I have accepted my fate but if I have learnt one thing it is that a problem understood by others who give support makes so much difference. It helps with the days of isolation I experienced in the early years. Then I was apparently a square peg that did not fit into any hole. It seemed absurd that I had something no one seemed to know anything about.

However, the fact still remains that my 'norm' is very painful."

"On a daily basis I am rarely without the crushing feeling of the fingers on my left hand. My fingers move incessantly in a clawing fashion against a strong pressure in my fingertips which in themselves feel bound by very tight elastic bands. The surface of my nails, which feel as though they are being pulled away from their attachments, have the appearance and feel of corrugated card and cannot tolerate any type of cosmetic painting to improve their appearance and trimming them is quite traumatic. They change from very hard and brittle to soft as tissue with no apparent reasoning and grow quite rapidly. The affected hand appears to me to look older and yet the appearance of 'age spots' is not as obvious as the other hand. Various warty-like lesions come and go."

"Relaxation, I understood, reduces pain, but for me, when I try, the opposite is the case. Any bodily stimulation, a candlelit, lazy bath, a nice swim or when travelling (and, as it happens, writing about it now) my fingers go into spasm and pound and certain digits become totally out of my control however hard I try. I am left with what feels like a 'club' on the end of my arm. This together with extreme sweating became apparent during various research applications. If I let my hand hang down beside me the pressure of tremendous weight builds and starts this 'club' syndrome I invariably hold on to the cuff of my clothing on that side to support my arm. I get very sharp stabbing pains in the wrist area but am now able to lift my arm above my head and turn my wrist some of the way round but not up and down to any extent. Often any pressure put on this hand results in a noise that sounds like bone snapping. My comfort zone is a quite contorted shape.

My fear is that my other hand and wrist are becoming painful."

This lady, so far, has found no means of relaxing.

Other techniques used for attention regulation and relaxation.

All other techniques employed use forms of relaxation called 'cognitive restructuring'. These are employed by psychologists and the details are outside the scope of this book, but put simply, involve establishing hierarchies, or orders of threats, and then attempting to teach desensitisation. They all try, with varying degrees of success, to disrupt the associations between pain, fear and tension that amplify pain. What do people tell us about these programmes?

Reactions are very mixed but where they are positive it is clear that the sufferer knows what it is all about and, where negative, think that someone is suggesting they are making it up or mad. Hopefully this book will have explained the importance of these programmes.

It is possible to do it yourself, but as in all things, a little bit of quality training helps. If the support you are given is inadequate shop around. The principles and effects are profound, but like medicine generally the practice is variable. If you are not prepared to try it and work at it thin it cannot work and your negative attitudes become self-fulfilling.

Biofeed-back and pain

Biofeedback is a treatment technique in which people are trained to improve their health by using signals from their own bodies. Relaxation therapies are a kind of biofeedback, but often not thought of as such. Biofeedback normally involves gadgets or machines that 'go ping'. The kind of kit that gets Monty Python and our head of medical physics, Dr. Nigel Harris over-excited.

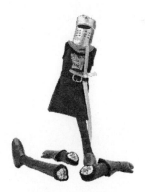

The hyper-excitable but persistent black knight, losing bodily control due to a lack of normal proprioceptive feedback.
From Monty Python.

Physical therapists use biofeedback to help stroke victims regain movement in paralyzed muscles. Using techniques, of varying degrees of sophistication, it has helped in chronic pain states where other treatments have failed. The principles are similar to those we have discussed, which are firstly, to shift attention away from the pain to a painless part of the body or something else, and to relax sufficiently to view pain as a neutral, not hurtful sensation. This technique, like others, aims to help the sufferer to try to regard pain as being of low intensity and try to gain control of the pain experience.

So what is it? You will recall that in one of the dialogues we describe a CRPS sufferer who could change the colour of her limb, but didn't know, or could not say, just how she pulled this trick. It would be beyond a normal person's capacity to change the blood flow to one limb at will. It clearly suggests that at least one part of the pain network is controllable by a near conscious cognitive process. One speculates if she can worsen it she may be able to do the opposite. If we produced a continuous real time thermo-graphic image of her limb, which she could see clearly and interpret immediately, she could then explore processes that may influence the blood supply.

Say, for example, she finds certain thoughts distressing and they stimulate her sympathetic system - the limb, being super sensitive to small changes, will change colour. Having done that we help her to do the opposite and explore those aspects fully. Now, armed with improvement images or metaphors she can incorporate these into her relaxation and programmed exercise activities. That is biofeedback. Thermography would be one way, but there are many others such as skin conductance.

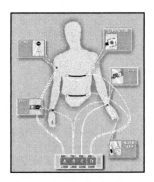

Biofeedback woman linked to all kinds of machines that go ping...
From home.iprimus.com.au/ rboon/Biofeedback.htm

Whilst this has been done successfully in chronic pain and something similar in migraine, it has not to our knowledge been done in CRPS. This technique is worthy of further attention. If any sufferer or carer has expertise in these areas we would like to assist them. We have a few ideas, but they may not be the best.

Help From Other Sufferers. The Expert Patient Programme

The Expert Patients Programme is a self-management course. It aims to giving people the confidence, skills and knowledge to manage their condition better and be more in control of their lives. It embraces pain suffers and also patients suffering from diseases such as cancer, heart disease, stroke and arthritis. Patient self-management or Expert Patient Programmes are based on developing patients' confidence and motivation and most of us could benefit from that.

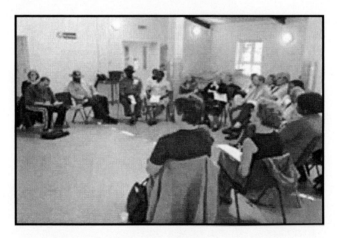

Patients on the Expert Patient Programme.

The purpose of these programmes is to provide 'effective control over life with a chronic condition'. The EPP course is based upon research over the past twenty years by a team led by Professor Kate Lorig at the Patient Education Research Centre, Stanford University, California. Within the UK, the Expert Patient Programme is based on courses and organized by the NHS.

These are run over six consecutive weekly sessions of 2.5 hours each week supported by two volunteer tutors. These are people with a chronic disease who lead 8-16 participants through structured course material delivered from a scripted manual.

This covers topics such as relaxation, diet, exercise, fatigue, breaking the symptom cycle, managing pain and medication, and communication with health care professionals. This is very similar to the format of this book as the attendees' recount their stories and others learn from them and advice. Many see their condition improve or stabilize.

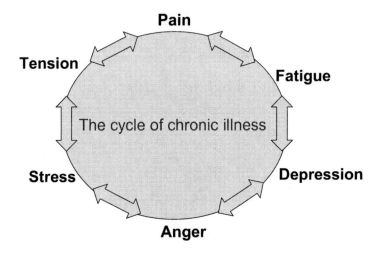

The basic aims of the EPP are to manage the cycle of chronic illness and medication more effectively through shared knowledge.

Participants on the course use a manual called 'Living a healthy life with chronic conditions'. This is based on a book used at Stanford University. It has been adapted for use in England. RSD-UK encourages suffers to attend and contribute. The following has been taken from the NHS expert patient web site.

Our hospital is contributing to the programmes.

"Are you a good listener? Are you motivated? Do you want to make a positive difference to the life of others? Become a course tutor and help others manage their long-term conditions.

Expert patients will:

- Feel confident and in control of their lives
- Aim to manage their condition and its treatment in partnership with health care professionals
- Communicate effectively with professionals and are wiling to share responsibility on treatment
- Are realistic about the impact of their disease on themselves and their family
- Use their skills and knowledge to lead full lives."

The Carer

Approximately 5.7million people in the UK care for a relative, friend, partner, or child with a disability. One adult in eight in the UK is a carer and nearly a quarter of carers have been doing so for at least 10 years. Many do not get support or training and are unaware that it is available and how important it is to seek it.

Being a good carer is considerably more difficult than being a good health professional.

It is, as the American's would say, a 24/24, 7/7, 52/52 job and hardly any are trained. In the UK we call this full-time!

A good carer makes all the difference in the world to a CRPS sufferer, a bad one can inadvertently do harm. The most common problem is not lack of caring, but over caring. This pushes the sufferer into the negative cycle of care. Here are the cycles. We list useful sources of information at the end of the book.

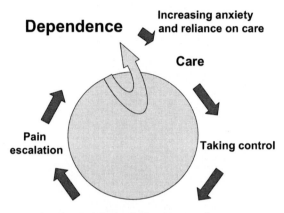

Getting it wrong

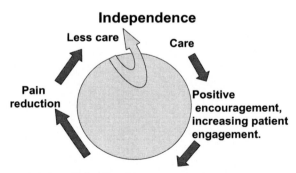

Drugs, but don't hold your breath

If there were a magic bullet that treated CRPS this book would not have been written.

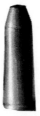

There are no magic bullets for CRPS

There are many pain relieving, analgesic medications, available. No one drug has shown a clear advantage in CRPS. Some work for a period but the effect seems to lessen with time. This is to be expected given the complex nature of the pain network. It is hard to imagine that drugs targeted to isolated pathways will confer long-lasting benefit. More block-buster drugs such as opiates come with many problems, and also are surprisingly ineffective for many. We describe a variety of drug types.

Be aware that many patients tell us that the drug didn't give benefit, but things worsened when they were stopped. This does not mean that they were working.

Drugs are merely a way of improving acceptance of physiotherapy programmes. They do not appear to have any curative qualities in this disease beyond that. If the drug does not help with mobilisation programmes and with sleep, reconsider it. The advice and comments given here are brief and certainly not comprehensive. They provide a general introduction to the area in order to help with discussions with your doctors. As we say, read the label, which is almost impossible in CRPS as the writing is far too small and for many will appear blurred. Make sure someone reads it to you.

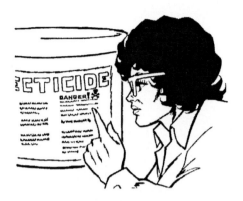

Read the label
www.subgenius.com

Opiates

Opiates are not generally considered an appropriate treatment for CRPS and should be taken with extreme reticence. They are powerful and from a doctor's perspective, flexible. It is perhaps surprising that their effect in CRPS appears marginal and this underlines the complexity of the pain network which is recruited in this syndrome. Most other pains are very sensitive to such drugs.

Opiates are any drug, natural or synthetic, that has morphine-like qualities. They are narcotics, meaning any substance that causes dependence. The word narcotic is derived from a Greek word meaning stupor. The body produces its own opiates called endorphins. Long-term use of opiates suppresses the formation of endorphins and disrupts the natural sleep pattern. The nocturnal sleep pattern is interrupted due to the known withdrawal phenomenon, leaving the sufferer tired during the day. The long- term use of morphine suppresses the immune system and many other systems.

Opiates can be sub-classified as weak or strong. An example of weak is codeine or propoxyphene; the rest are strong. Opiates react to cause their effects through molecules on cells that dock with them. These are known as receptors. There are six different receptors and they are found throughout the body. These guarantee some unwanted effects which are not to be confused with allergic effects.

174

One of the most common, unwanted effects of morphine and other opiates including dihydrocodeine is constipation and it does not get better with time, but assistance can be given. There are a variety of other unwanted problems.

The concern over addiction is lessening as available evidence shows clearly that this occurs rarely if prescribed for pain in patients with no previous addiction or drug abuse problems. This is surprising, but has been found many times in research studies.

A side effect occurs in a proportion of people taking a drug; it may be unwanted or allergic.
An unwanted effect occurs in many, albeit to varying degrees.
"Morphine made me constipated", is an unwanted side effect.

An allergic reaction is a side effect caused by a specific allergic immune reaction.

"Penicillin caused my body to swell and I could barely breathe," is an allergic side effect.

Opiates nevertheless have a small part to play in CRPS management if other drugs have failed. The guidelines for use have been established. Firstly, the reason for prescribing them needs to be defined clearly and the best is short-term help with physiotherapy compliance. However, if the regimes described above are fulfilled in a timely fashion, opiates will be needed in a small fraction of the CRPS population. Next, a short trial should be undertaken to make sure these objectives are achieved and unwanted effects are dealt with. Sometimes, in a hospital setting, a short-acting intravenous compound is used for this purpose. The optimal dose needs to be established. Doctors will avoid the drugs that have a very rapid effect, as these tend to lead to more abuse problems. Carers need to partake in the process as they need to keep a careful look out for misuse. If all this sounds 'nannyish' it is because one disease is bad enough and opiate abuse creates many more difficulties. On the other side of the coin, there is no need to be "opiophobic" and pain does need treatment. Opiates can improve the quality of some people's lives. Nevertheless, we stress again that CRPS pain does not as a general rule, respond well to opiates. Some of our patients take methadone, used primarily for heroin addiction; in general it does not impair cognitive functions.

There are lots of other drugs for allodynic (neuropathic) diseases. No drug has been found to have an indisputable effect in modern trials but plenty have been found to have an influence anecdotally.

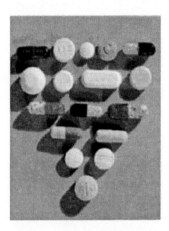

Choice is difficult, individual and unpredictable. Red tablets have the best placebo effect and blue the worst in most studies.

You need a lot of patients to do a trial and few centres see anything like enough people to establish a trial to the standards required by a drug licensing authority. In addition, as CRPS is not a big market for pharmaceutical studies, they do not initiate trials frequently and clinical trials are very expensive. All drugs listed are the proper names and not the companies' licensed name which varies between companies and in different countries. For instance Paracetamol and Tylenol are the same - acetaminophen.

Simple over-the-counter medications for pain such as acetaminophen and aspirin derivatives, of which there are many, do little to help the pains we have described. However, some drugs developed to treat epilepsy (anticonvulsants), depression (antidepressants) and unstable heart rhythms (antiarrythmics) surprisingly do, a bit...sometimes. There is no clear leader and informed trial and error is the only approach. This is perhaps best undertaken by a hospital-based pain specialist who will have much greater familiarity with these drugs. The pain specialist will also appreciate the importance of using drugs as part of a package of care delivered by the pain team. Do not accept drugs from someone who is saying, in effect, "take these drugs and I don't need to see you again, your GP will cope.

Anticonvulsants

There is a bias towards using these drugs for the lancing-type pains that are so common and very troublesome. This prejudice does not have a secure scientific foundation and is based on individual patient observations. The drugs that have been used include phenytoin, carbamezepine, sodium valproate, lamotrigine, gabapentin and a new gabapentinoid, pregabalin. These drugs have been shown to have an effect, to varying degrees, in diseases where nerves degenerate and release neuropeptides which cause pain and open blood vessels. Some work in viral neuropathies such as herpes. Others work in pain that follows certain strokes and in migraine. For each drug the allergic, unwanted and side effect profile varies. Certain medical conditions prevent their use.

Antidepressants

The bias here is towards the burning pains so often mentioned in the dialogues and again a major cause of suffering. Three different classes of antidepressants have been used in neuropathic pain states as a whole. These include tricyclic antidepressants, and selective uptake inhibitors. The latter includes selective serotonin reuptake agents such as paroxetine, citalopram, fluoxetine, and sertraline.

Venlaflaxine also blocks a compound released after stimulation of the autonomic nervous system noradrenalin (norepinephrine). Tricyclic antidepressants have the most published data to support their use in neuropathic pain states generally, but even here where the evidence is best, two or three patients need to be treated to find one whose pain is reduced by half compared to placebo. These tricyclics include drugs such as imipramine, amitryptilene, clomipramine, desipramine, nortryptilene, mirtazapine, and maprotilene. Again, certain medical conditions limit their use including glaucoma, some heart problems and convulsive disorders.

Side effects and unwanted effects are very common and many cannot obtain an analgesic response before they occur. Some are helpful to aid sleep in lower doses. Most patients with CRPS have tried these agents.

Antiarrhyhmics

A cardiac drug, mexilitene, has been used in certain neuropathic diseases. Unlike many of the drugs in this group it can be taken by mouth. You need to treat ten patients to find one who responds by fifty percent. This is one for the specialist only.

Other drugs tried

Corticosteroids may provide relief in CRPS, but their long-term use is not recommended. Other agents that have received limited clinical use in CRPS include clonidine, ketamine, muscle relaxants, sympatholytic drugs (e.g., prazosin), calcium channel blockers, and baclofen, but data on their relative efficacy is lacking. Topical capsaicin is unlikely to offer great benefit.

More hopeful news is a class of drugs routinely used to treat osteoporosis. You will recall that transient osteoporosis is a short- term feature of some patients. The drugs belong to the bisphosphonate family, and bind permanently to the surfaces of the bones and slow down bone-eroding cells.

This allows the bone-building cells to work more effectively. One drug, Pamidronate, may be a useful treatment option in the management of patients with CRPS Type I. The treatment response was variable, but the majority of patients improved.

Early administration in tandem with other treatment measures is recommended. This seems safe and worthy of much further study. The pain relieving effects are not easily explained by what we know of the drug's action at this stage.

Blocking the sympathetic system

The sympathetic system was once quite commonly blocked both for therapeutic and diagnostic use. It is now less commonly done and the therapeutic advantages seriously questioned. One reason for not doing it is that sympathetically maintained pain is a short-lived and fluctuating phenomenon and other parts of the network supervene to maintain the pain process. In groups where it was done therapeutically only a third showed any effect after multiple invasive blocks. It rarely lasts for long.

We have been unimpressed by the short and long-term benefits and have little enthusiasm for the procedure. Others do not share this view. There are a variety of different ways of blocking the sympathetic chain. The safest, probably, is with local anaesthetic agents or a 'regional block' with a drug called guanethidine. This is done with a limb tourniquet. Some of the other procedures including ablation by radio waves, certain destructive chemicals (neurolytic drugs) or surgery can produce new allodynic symptoms.

Hyperbaric Oxygen

Patients with a wide range of diseases have been treated with oxygen delivered at high pressure for at least two hundred years. It has been advocated, again with sparse evidence, to be effective in some CRPS patients. We have little experience and our comments are similar to those stated above.

Most comments on the web are difficult to interpret, but generally show enthusiasm. It is relatively easy to measure the extent of the disease both in terms of symptoms and signs using a host of quantitative test systems and the lack of such data from centres with experience is of concern.

Other non drug non physiotherapy based treatments

Spinal cord simulation

It is possible to insert electrodes around the spinal cord and influence pain signalling networks. The procedure can be done by pain specialists inserting electrodes through the skin and into a space around the cord known as the epidural space. It is the same place anaesthetist use for certain regional anaesthesia procedures. Patients can control the amount of stimulation via a box.

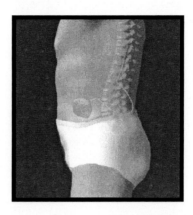

Spinal cord stimulation - from the International Research Foundation for RSD/CRPS who provide more extensive details.

Please see rsdfoundation.org

How well does it work? Most reported studies seem enthusiastic and recommend early treatment. The quality of the evidence is limited and others reporting are less enthusiastic. We have no experience and therefore do not comment or expand further.

It would be helpful for future editions of this book to obtain feedback from those who have had the procedure. Doctors and scientists, when describing limited trial series on selected people, are biased towards publishing the data if it is positive. Patients responding to requests like this are more likely to do so if they have a 'bad news' story. Please let us know either way. It would be useful to know if it works best early or late. In practice it is mainly used late in the disease. It has been used during pregnancy with a good effect reported and no harm to the foetus.

Electro-Convulsive Therapy- ECT

Cases have been presented in the scientific literature, describing electroconvulsive therapy for depression associated with CRPS. ECT led to the relief of CRPS as well as depression. In one of the cases concomitant fibromyalgia, another chronic pain disease, was not relieved. Another neuropathic pain state trigeminal neuralgia has responded.

It is stated that the pain relieving effects of ECT are not only due to improving depression, it appears to work directly on a part of the pain network. Again, we ask if anyone has experience, to let us know.

Electro-Convulsive Therapy has received bad press, mainly based on its previous use without adequate anaesthetics and muscle relaxants. ECT is an electric shock delivered to the brain which produces fits or seizures in the person receiving it. It is usually given 3 times a week. A patient may require as few as 3 or 4 treatments or as many as 12 to 15. Today the method is painless. The statistical risk of dying from receiving ECT is roughly 4 in 100,000. It has been estimated that there are around 138,000 treatments a year in Britain. We cannot recommend it, other than an option of last resort, but we may be being too cautious. It is a shame that the reports of its use in CRPS lack the detail needed to make a clear assessment.

Genetics and inheritance

At our clinic we have seen identical twins, middle aged women, who had both recently developed CRPS following minimal trauma. Is this coincidence or the influence of genes? Others have looked at this and one study reported on the Web, "In our series of 386 consecutive patients diagnosed as suffering from RSD, only 4 families (with more than one member of the family suffering from RSD) were identified." This would seem to the authors of this book to be an enhanced risk over chance alone and suggest an inheritable contribution. It is however a complex issue the authors of the original text didn't think much of it.

We are regularly asked, "Is this disease inherited, or are my children at risk"? The answer is not clear-cut. We need to explain more, and Mr and Mrs Man in the street's understanding of modern genetics is often not so good. We therefore start at the beginning. Put up with us if you live in 'an avenue' and know all this.

My son looks a bit like me and like his mum is kind, and works hard probably because of her too. This is because he has inherited traits from both of us and in passing our traits we are giving him hereditable features. My other son is a plonker and so was the milk man. Our traits come from our genes, rarely just one, more often a combination.

Our genes live on our DNA which is packaged in chromosomes inside the nucleus of our cells. The environment may influence our traits, so my son may actually be a plonker because peer pressure at school disrupted his education. He may come good later in a different environment.

We each have two sets of twenty three chromosomes giving us forty six in all. Sperm and eggs have one set of chromosomes each. When we mix these two and conceive a child we each give one complete set to the child. A woman has two X chromosomes making her a female (XX) and a man an X and a Y making him a fellow (XY). Each parent contributes one set, but any individual chromosome comes randomly from either of the two sets. So far so good.

Here is a diagram to show one nuclear family, Adam and Eve with two kids, and for simplicity we are only giving them 5 chromosomes per set, but remember there are in fact 23. Adam is the XY, male and Eve the XX female.

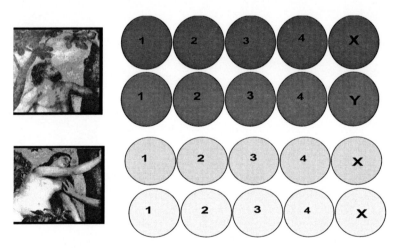

Now Adam and Eve had three sons and maybe daughters which we did not hear about. Here are two of the lads, two brothers, but plenty of genetic differences, and we only showed five chromosomes so with twenty three they would be considerably different.

182

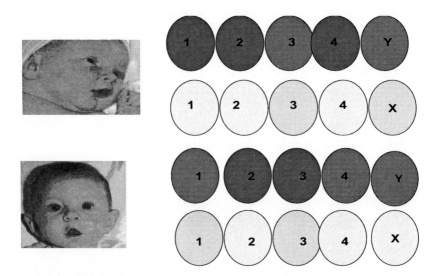

On each of the chromosomes are multiple genes and genes function as instruction guides for protein production. Proteins do many things; some are enzymes driving chemical reactions.

Genes are attached to DNA strands. Whilst the process of operating our 25,000 genes is complex it is certain to falter some time. When a gene goes faulty the protein it produces may be mutated and disease may be a consequence. Many genes are linked together producing sets of proteins working together on a complex task. The amount of variety that can be generated by mutated proteins is unbelievable. Some mutations are lethal, some are beneficial and nature and evolution depend upon this.

Genes may affect the onset of a disease, or how it progresses and in what form. Genes can influence us by their actions or inactions. An absence of a gene may be the cause of an event if the protein it produced functioned as a negative controller.

Now you see that the question "Is CRPS inherited?" is complex. Firstly, do you mean can it be inherited? Probably. Do you mean how likely it to be inherited is? Not very. Or if I hurt myself could genes be the reason I overespond? Almost certainly. CRPS may not be a disease in a classical sense, but a massively amplified intrinsically normal pain response. It could be because there is too much of a positive feedback system or too little of a negative one. Each component could be inherited and there may be many positive and negative points of control.

We have 25,000 genes.
A roundworm has 19,000 genes,
and a fruit fly 13,601 genes.

The difference between mammalian genes is important. Most genes are conserved among mammals however we are distinct from our evolutionary relatives.

What makes us human? This question has useful medical applications.

For example, which mammals do not get cancer? Which mammals cannot catch acquired immune deficiency syndrome (AIDS)? What animals do or do not get CRPS? What is it about their immune/inflammatory systems and bodily make-up that makes them more or less resilient than us?

Understanding how genes have evolved in different species may help us develop of better drugs and therapies for humans and other species.

We do know that women have this disease more often than men suggesting some effect of the X chromosome or some protective effect of the Y. This suggests a genetic influence of the sex chromosomes in part. Is that due to hormones or another feature found on the X chromosome or a control feature of the Y? The hippocampus as we have described is oestrogen, a female hormone, sensitive.
In fact, as far as we can tell all diseases have some genetic input; it seems to be a factor in influencing about one quarter or a third of the process. The cause of CRPS is trauma of some kind, or at least fine nerve damage. This occurs all the time, therefore the influence of genes is probably not as a pure cause, but as a means of influencing if, when and how problems will come to light.

Of course, asking does anyone else in the family have RSD/CRPS is one question, but asking does anyone have a disease such as these in the table, quite another. You will by now understand why we have chosen these. From this kind of question we may identify clustering of diseases and get a much clearer understanding of key genetic mechanisms. We presently have weak anecdotal evidence that these diseases do cluster in some families, but we are not certain how much more likely than by chance alone.

But this is also true…

"My own experience suggests that any genetic element is likely to be weak, since my brother, my sister and two of my sons each broke an arm at some stage and never developed RSD. I went through childhood and brought up a family without breaking a limb, despite many falls but, when I did eventually break my arm, I quickly developed RSD. From the evidence to date there seems to be **no reason to worry**. Derrick Phillips - Editor of RSD Alert"

Does CRPS have a purpose?

Aristotle spent considerable time during his life trying to understand how we define things. Not some things, but all things. He came up with series of clauses as a structure. They hold good to this day and are a good place to start when trying to tackle complex problems. Here is an example. What is a kitchen spoon?

It is an object with a characteristic shape. [CRPS is a syndrome with a characteristic pattern of signs and symptoms.]

It is made of steel a combination of iron and carbon of variable ratios. [CRPS is a disease generated by central drivers and peripheral outputs of variable molecular and electrical composition.] Now if that's all you knew you wouldn't know much until we discussed its purpose to get foods to your mouth. So what's the purpose of CRPS? It is most definitely not to make you a better person through suffering or to punish you for previous generation's sins; ideas that are occasionally generated by religion- cf AIDS.

Genetics Questionnaire

Does anybody in your genetic family have, or has had, one of these diseases

CRPS

Anorexia or similar

Migraine

Epilepsy

Dystonia

(Autism)

We hold to certain genetic predisposition because sometime back they gave primitive man or his ancestors a survival advantage. So now a bit of speculation based on this model. Why do we have so many people in the western world who get diabetes and high cholesterol? The answer is in a society where food is sparse hanging on to sugars and fat longer keep you reduce the risk of starvation induced death. So the fast metabolises die off and the slow live longer and breed more. This explains why the surviving descendents of slaves are prone to these problems and suffer when exposed to high sugar and fat convenience foods. To understand CRPS we need to go further back than a few generations and to different species. Consider this rabbit alive and in a trap and now consider a primitive rabbit with a leg trapped by natural circumstances.

In these circumstances the rabbit who can self amputate his limb will survive longer than the one that can't. Some more primitive species like the gecko can self amputate to minimal trauma or the threat of it. They can regenerate a limb. Neither the rabbit nor we can.

Now consider the symptoms and signs of CRPS in this light and remember the rabbit may well feel the pain somewhat differently. The peripheral inflammation is a great sterilisation system, the neglect an

186

alien felling allow you to get the courage to self amputate and rabbits can gnaw off their limbs under these extreme circumstances. Their survival chances are not good but better than nil if nothing or no other rabbit can help. This is known as an autotomy reaction. It may be a primitive explanation of purpose. You maybe able to think of better theoretical models.

Much more to say, but time to stop

We have covered most of the important symptoms and signs that define the syndrome. We have explored the negative and to some extent the positive cognitive consequences.

We have done our best to put this into a scientific context and described treatment programmes that follow. There is a long way to go and much more research to be done, not least in the field of genetics.

We leave our final words to the founder of RSD UK who has achieved an enormous amount and taught and inspired us all.

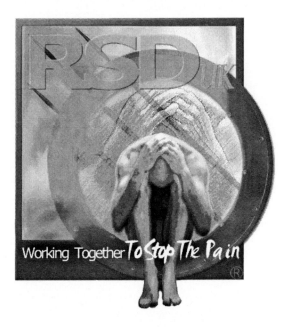

RSD UK, the charity, written by Catherine Taylor

"RSD UK started its journey in September 2000 after I realised no structured support for patients with this condition was available; the charity is still run by the two founding members, me and Barry Swallow. Before I go further, on behalf of all our members I would like to thank

Barry for his dedicated work behind the scenes; without this hard work RSD UK would shudder to a halt.

RSD UK is the registered UK Charity for those interested in Reflex Sympathetic Dystrophy/Complex Regional Pain Syndrome. By 'interested' we mean patients and their family, friends and carers, medical professionals and the occasional curious journalist. RSD UK has over 1500 patients on the member database; we think there are around 11,600 patients in the UK. We are therefore striving to find ways to reach more of the RSD/CRPS population.

It is said there are an estimated 1.5 million suffers in the USA. Given the population of the USA is 296 million and there are 60 million in the UK, which is roughly five times less, there should be 300,000 in the UK. This is a lot more than our estimate of 11,600. Reasons please, but sufferers from the USA and of course other nationals are very welcome to access our site and to contribute to this book.

So, what do we do at RSD UK? In short we try to help those patients having difficulty with the condition or who are having problems accessing appropriate medical treatment. We act as a buffer for the frustrations that occur with the battle to get recognition, understanding and treatment. We can be seen as a safety valve for patients who find it almost impossible cope with the condition. But that still doesn't answer the question "what do we do?"

There is no typical day. There is no typical telephone call. There are, however, typical scenarios patients relate to us by phone or in our forum.

"Can you help? I had Sudecks Atrophy, when I saw another doctor he said I had Causalgia too. I have also been diagnosed with RSD and the physiotherapist said I have got CRPS"

This lady thought she had a whole host of weird medical conditions; the sigh of relief was audible after explaining they are the same condition but holding an impressive plethora of titles!

And, here starteth the problems!

"My Orthopaedic Surgeon said I would be better in a few months but my Pain Doctor said I will never get better..."

How do we know who to believe?

If an Orthopaedic Surgeon sees this condition he is of the opinion that it 'burns itself out' it gets better in months or is the sign of an awkward patient. If a Consultant Anaesthetist or Rheumatologist sees the condition he is of the opinion that it is a disabling condition whereby the patient may never work again.

Are these generalisations? We think not. Which do we believe? The answer is simple – both of them! Doctors base their opinion on experience and understanding of a condition. In the case of our Orthopaedic Surgeon he may see numerous cases of early or minor RSD/CRPS, their trauma heals, they are discharged from his care and they never return – so the patient *must* have got better; and in many cases they have.

Our Consultant Anaesthetist or Rheumatologist however will usually be presented with the chronic, difficult to treat patient who has a noticeable disability due to the condition. He rarely sees the cases that resolve or are manageable as these patients are not referred to his clinic. So, his opinion that it is a disabling life-long condition is correct, based on the patients he sees.

Confused? This is one of the basics that callers question when contacting us via the helpline (0845 22 66 008).

Most callers have never had the condition explained to them in a way they can understand and this adds to the fear factor. We try to explain why the patient feels as they do in layman's terms, giving opportunity for questions where needed.

Taking calls from distraught patients raises mixed emotions from those taking the call; those making the calls are often confused, frightened, and unsure, isolated and may be disbelieved by family, friends and medical professionals.

For many, the call is the first time they have spoken to anyone who understands the condition; this can be overwhelming for the patient – to finally be believed without question. They chat freely about their bizarre symptoms and on hearing these are 'normal' they gain a sense of relief – they are not going crazy after all!

Sometimes the calls take a turn that couldn't be anticipated...

"Is that Catherine?"

"Yes, good morning, how can I help?"

There was uncontrollable sobbing for a few minutes; it is the type of call that leaves me feeling helpless. When the caller managed to speak the call was not what I was expecting.

"I am a GP and have ...had a patient with RSD." I let him take his time..."She has just committed suicide because we couldn't help her."

The GP was blaming himself; he was convinced he had let her and her young family down, he was inconsolable. His patient was married with 2 children under the age of 5 years old. Later that day the young woman's husband phoned. Although distraught he had nothing but praise for the medical profession and how they had tried to help; he held his GP in high esteem and felt guilty that the GP was blaming himself.

The reason I include this is because as patients we often fail to think about the impact that our condition has on our health care team. We become angry at the very people that are trying to help us. During your RSD/CRPS career you will meet many professionals who have no experience or knowledge of this condition until the day you turn up at their door. Their lack of experience/knowledge doesn't mean they are a 'bad doctor' - it means they haven't met the condition before. They are on a learning curve; they may look to you for answers. Thankfully most GP's are willing to learn but we still come across those who don't understand the condition and refuse to take time to learn; sometimes this unwillingness is coupled with an attitude that puts the 'blame' on the patient for a condition that the doctor does not understand.

Apart from direct contact with patients we liaise with many other agencies from research centres to governmental departments and charities involved in pain services. Where possible we work alongside other organizations for the benefit of our members and future patients.
We organise the sending out of patient information brochures and other literature, try to put patients in touch with other patients and organise the UK National RSD/CRPS Conference.

Barry works tirelessly sending out information brochures, keeping the database updated and arranging all but the speakers at the National Conference. He also has endless amounts of encouragement when the work gets a bit challenging!

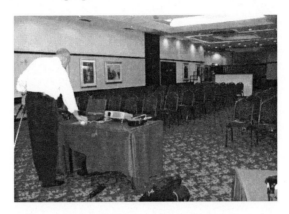

Barry started to worry when everyone left during his speech!

We endeavour to make our services accessible to all which means we receive letters, emails, and telephone calls and regulate the online forum; all these services are free of charge for the users and for the benefit of the patient. Details are displayed at the end of this book.

Another memorable call came from a young lady who is a wheelchair user who has locked joints:

"Hi Catherine, its Amy." "Hey, Amy, how are you?"

"Yeah, I'm good; I just did something quite mad"

"Oh yes? What was that?"

"I did a sponsored walk for RSD UK."

… And yes, she did mean walk! She braved the pain, donned her crutches and walked 1 mile to raise awareness and funds! RSD UK membership has a good scattering of Amy's, such as Malcolm Blackburn from Yorkshire who has raised around £5,000 in a 2 or 3 years!

192

Life is never dull at RSD UK – it is often distressing - but elating, tiring - but invigorating though more often than not the heartfelt "thank you" at the end of the call makes it all worthwhile.

And a poem like this makes all the hard work worthwhile. Thank you, Sue."

Today I Danced with my Daughter

For Rosie

Today I danced with my daughter.
I danced with her courage
And her pain
And her being-in-a-body
That will not respond to her wishes.

I danced the only willing parts of her body
That would yield and join our dance:
I danced her eyes,
And her eyelids,
And her lips that danced in smiles
Where an absence of smiles
Would be forgiven.

And as I danced her spirit
- Blessed that I was to be shown it flying free –
I coaxed and cajoled reluctant muscles
I sweet-talked stubborn sinews
And I begged her obstinate bones to move.

I asked those fingers that once played piano,
Those legs that used to run,
The belly that used to laugh
And those shoulders that used to sway
As they carried the heavily scented songs of her alto sax
To dance, to dance.
To dance.

And when they wouldn't

And when they couldn't
I danced her exasperation and her sorrow and her anger
Which fast became my own;
A rage twisting its way up from where it had been held,
Unsuspected in my spine.
A rage that thrashed its way through me,
Vertebra by vertebra,
A spooked horse foaming,
As it crashed its way roaring,
Through a course
Of splintered jumps.
And I wanted to take my daughter
By her stupid stubborn shoulders
And shake shake shake them
And make make make them move
Until the folly of it and uselessness of it and the frustration of it
Gave way to a grief
Lying heavy in my hips,
So pregnant with unformed fears it felt
As though
I had lost my baby.

Today I danced with my daughter
Because I had to dance that dance:
Its power was so big,
So staggeringly huge,
It was too vast for me to hold
In the spaces between my own set of bones.
And had it not been danced
It would have weighed me down, seducing,
A stagnant monster swamp
Swelling and sucking me
Down to drown
In inertia's boggy grief.

Today I danced with my daughter
As she lay, unmoving,
In her clinical hospital bed.
And I wept.

Su Hughes 2005

194

The Epilogue

The Story Teller's Story

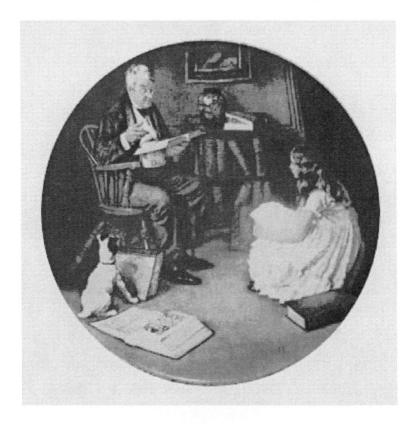

The Story Teller
From theplatelady.com/ normanrockwell/story-teller

It has been said that "ill people are more than victims of disease or patients of medicine; they are wounded storytellers", the author, whose details are in the reference list, argues. People tell stories to make sense of their suffering; when they turn their diseases into stories, they find healing. In a book written by Arthur Frank, he tells a stirring collection of illness narratives, of people with cancer, chronic fatigue syndrome, and disabilities. Critics suggest the stories are more than accounts of personal suffering and embrace moral choices and point to a social ethic. The author identifies three basic narratives of illness - stories of restitution, chaos, and quest. "Restitution narratives anticipate getting well and give prominence to the technology of cure. In chaos narratives, illness seems to stretch on forever, with no respite or redeeming insights. Quest narratives are about finding that illness can be transformed into a means for the ill person to become someone new. Understanding these three narrative types helps us to hear the ill, but ultimately illness stories are more. Frank presents these stories as a form of testimony: the ill person is more than a survivor; she is a witness. Schooled in 'pedagogy of suffering', the ill person reaches out to others, offering a truth about living. The truth is a starting point for a 'narrative ethics', as private experiences become public voices. Wounded storytellers teach more than a new way to understand illness; they exemplify an emerging ethic of post-modern times."

Fancy writing, but clear enough. We see our lives, and parts of it, as stories where we are beset in illness by dragons which we or others may defeat. We are the suffering princess looking for a prince who may not come in the form of modern medicine.

We choose to end this book with a story of suffering and allodynic pain, told by one of the authors as 'his story,' though he was not the sufferer, the princess, or indeed the prince that slays the dragon; merely the story teller.

The story of the crown versus Dr. Nigel Cox. A story about allodynia and suffering

"This is a story that is based upon my recollection of a trial for murder, or a variant of murder, called man-slaughter. If you are found guilty of manslaughter the punishment is discretionary.

As it happens, due to ignorance of the law, I had no idea of this until I was called as an expert witness to defend Nigel. I had kept as far away from the law as possible, it seemed an organisation so monstrously large and tortuous that only a fool would not fear it.

Dr Cox is probably my best friend-friend. I have a lot of acquaintance-friends, but these are of little use if you are in trouble. Most of us judge our friends by their admirable qualities. This strikes me as a daft idea as admirable qualities have a habit of being illusionary. It can take an age before you discover this, as CRPS suffers know only to well.
I measure true friendships in terms of units of distance that the friend would travel to help you if in great trouble. I use an old fashioned imperial scale, inches feet yards or miles. Nigel is a 10,000 mile friend despite being profoundly irritating. His admirable qualities are few, but certainly not illusionary. He is loyal, stubborn and a first rate doctor. Most acquaintances are inches, feet or yard 'friends'.

What makes a good doctor? Not charm, not sophistication; these are admirable all right, but not enough. A good doctor admits it to himself and the patient when he does not know what is going on and asks another for advice. He continues to do this until he is sure he has the best advice. He does not refer passively for an opinion; he is active in his search for one. There are many admirable doctors but very few good ones.

Nigel phones me about once a fortnight to ask me about someone or tell me about someone, which is much the same thing. He wants to know if I agree. I phone Nigel about once in three months. Now you may think that's because I am a professor and therefore clever and Nigel is just your bog-standard hospital doctor who works outside our great University institutions.

Nigel does not phone me because he is stupid. He phones me because he is a generalist and deals with many diseases and I'm a specialist dealing with very few. I can keep up with my field, he can't and he really would be daft if he thought he could.

So now I need to tell you a story about specialisation and specialists, and people like me.

"I returned from school, clutching a sealed report that I had opened, which said 'could do better'. This I understood, aged fourteen, to be bad. It also added, 'Suffers fools badly' which seemed to me a compliment.

My mother read the report handed it back to me and told me this was my father's business. He read the report, said nothing and went to his book case and handed me two books. The first was small and entitled 'The Specialist' and the second a novel entitled 'The Revolt of Gunner Ash'.

"Read them", was all he said. So I did, and told him so. "Read them again" he said, "and make notes, and work out what they mean, and why I gave them to you. Your report, I might add, suggests you're bright, but not bright enough, you are intolerant of institutions and some of the people in them."

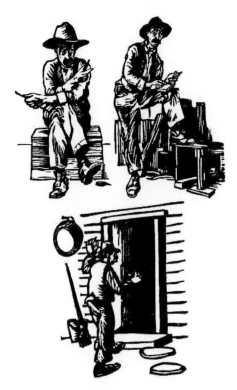

'The Specialist'. By Charles Sayle.

CRPS is easy to diagnose by a specialist, not easy for a generalist.

Now what is in these books is crucial to the whole plot: Not only of this story, but the book as a whole.

Gunner Asch is a perfectly solid bloke, with qualities that are admirable and not illusionary. To help his close friends he would travel far. He is conscripted into the German Army and eventually finds himself in 1943 on the Eastern front, which is precisely where you would not want to be. Gunner Asch is surrounded both above and below in the Weirmacht by an enormous number of people. They represent every variant or deviant our genes can generate and then the environment modify. Gunner Asch has to survive a war that is inevitably lost, but ensure that as many of his immediate circle, of friend-friends and friend-acquaintances, do as well. In addition, being a decent human being, he also helps a few intolerables from the far right and far left of this bunch. How he achieves this is portrayed with considerable humour and the book was easy even for a kid of fourteen, who had not as yet set his mind to great philosophical thoughts.

Now 'The Specialist' is also humorous and far more subtle. The book is short, taking an hour or so to read, but tells you all you need to know to be a specialist. The key character in this American novelette is a man called Len Putt who was a general carpenter until he studied 'specialism'.

He knew immediately that was the way to go. It's easy; secondly you get to 'feeling proud'. Len Putt specialised in outdoor lavatories or 'privies' as he called them, "and damn fine privies they were too, with hearts in the door for the women and square holes as seats for the farm labourers to sit on, with rough edges so they didn't tarry too long". Now that's 'specialism'.

My father read my notes and said," What do you want to be when you grow up?" I said "I wanted to be a specialist carpenter and work alone... and avoid institutions and bigots and stuff."

And my father said "You are not bright enough, practical enough and without any inherent business skills so you are going to be a 'specialist', a consultant, and work for the NHS" and I thought "It's better than the army" and kept my mouth shut... which cheered up my father no end.

So that's how I came to defend Nigel as a specialist and why Nigel wanted me to, and the defence thought I could too… because though I'm no Gunner Asch, I can do it for an hour or two.

So now we go to court. A crown court, which is where they try you in front of a jury to see if you're 'mad, sad, bad, sick, thick or a....'. Which is how lawyers assess us and doctors assess patients, though we all keep it to ourselves.

We start with Nigel's patient and subsequent victim, who was not known to me during her life. Later I met her family and some of her many friends. Her story is available on the web though to my mind it is as we say 'half cocked'. Lillian Boyce had severe rheumatoid arthritis with a variety of unusual life threatening complications that had caused unimaginable pain and suffering for years.

I will not dwell on the details, but when an unavoidable bed sore penetrated through her back and into her bowel she decided to refuse all further treatment. The consequence of this had to be death within a few weeks to a few months. She involved her family and friends in her decision to be certain that her actions caused the minimum of anguish. They agreed with her. She informed Nigel who she knew well and respected. He had pulled her through many a medical crisis in the past and they too were friends. He was reluctant, but following many discussions with Lillian and her family he concurred, albeit reluctantly.

Mrs. Boyce was to stay on her painkillers and stop all other medication that was sustaining her life. These included steroids. The abrupt withdrawal of steroids in someone who has needed them for years causes 'adrenal failure' which is life threatening. In Lillian's case not a possibility, a certainty.

Her health detonated rapidly and her pain worsened. He prescribed morphine in increasing amounts and this would be judged appropriate by his peers and the law. He was obliged to increase the dose to one that would of itself shorten life and this is acceptable to our profession and the law.

Then, and I recall from memory the description of a nurse at the trial for manslaughter. "Lillian would cry like… I don't know… it was horrible… like someone had stood on a cat's foot…It was sickening."

200

This sounds like the description of an allodynic response. She was asked what would set it off "noise, any noise, a door closing, we tried to be so quiet, but you can't stop noise in hospital even in her own room". An increased prescription of morphine very unusually worsened the situation. (This is a very rare occurrence.) The relatives were distraught; Lillian, deeply unconscious, would scream in apparent pain to stimuli, but was otherwise comatose.

Nigel distraught, took an ampoule of potassium from the secure drugs cabinet, injected it intravenously and Lillian was at peace. Potassium causes cardiac arrest.

The case rested on the distinction between his motive and his intent.

The jury spent two days before failing to deliver a verdict. They returned and asked if I could repeat my evidence. The judge ruled this inappropriate, but said he would summarise.

Professor Blake said, "Intravenous potassium would certainly kill Lillian and agreed that any doctor would know that. When asked if potassium had any pain relieving properties, he replied no. "When asked by the prosecution if he would have given Mrs. Boyce potassium he replied, no."

The remaining two hours supportive testimony was omitted.

"I would remind that a jury does not pass sentence. It determines if the law of the land is broken. Did the doctor intend to kill Mrs. Boyce?"

The jury retired… and returned, some in tears, others close. The foreman and the jury avoided looking at the hushed courtroom. The foreman did well to make his response to the judges request clear.

The verdict was delivered. The court was silent, and then a frail old voice from the gallery said, "What they say, what they say?" And a kind voice said, "They said guilty, Mrs Cox" and Nigel's mum cried and Lillian's family cried, even the crown prosecutor cried…and the judge said we could take Nigel home so we did. It was, however, clear to most that though Nigel was, to put it bluntly, "as guilty of being an idiot, he was not guilty of murder… and we are all idiots from time to time, are we not?

A few days later Nigel was given a 'two year suspended sentence'. He was referred to our medical licensing body. He was found guilty of misconduct and asked to attend a pain training programme. It was pretty clear that despite the stern warning to Nigel and our profession in general, that they thought that even an idiot could be a pretty good doctor, if he had something else going for him.

Now let's leave the court, which is an unholy place despite the bibles you get to hold when telling them that you won't lie, but get as close to it as you possibly can... Mr. Clinton!"

This is the end of the story. It has princes and princesses and dragons, and is a tragedy where all ends well, but it took some effort by all the characters. CRPS is the same.

All the best.
DRB April 2006

A few useful web sites

RSD UK   [Rating *****] www.rsd-crps.co.uk
Awareness, Education and Support and a lot more

Reflex Sympathetic Dystrophy Association of America www.rsds.org
Information site. Promotes great awareness for Reflex Sympathetic
Dystrophy. Includes video, news clips and links.

Canadian Reflex Sympathetic Dystrophy Network www.canadianrsd.com
Good source of material

Arthritis Research Campaign (ARC) www.arc.org.uk
Raises funds to promote medical research into the cause, treatment and
cure of arthritic conditions including CRPS. Good educational material.
Funds key research programmes.

British Psychological Society www.bps.org.uk

And many others

Follow the links or type RSD and or CRPS on a search engine for quality
scientific papers use Google scholar's home page and key in the key
words we have used in the text ;for example CRPS and neglect or CRPS
and anger. Avoid commercial sites with advertisements is a good general
rule for unbiased information. If you are buying a product for CRPS
check with others who use the chat rooms or e mail services of the major
charities.

Useful Books on pain and phantoms available from Amazon. Com

Pain: The science of Suffering
by Patrick Wall. A very readable book. Our book is a sequel written as a
tribute to probably the supreme investigator of pain who died recently.

The Challenge of Pain (Penguin Science)
by Ronald Melzack, Patrick D. Wall. Also very readable.

Phantoms in the Brain: Probing the Mysteries of the Human Mind by V. S. Ramachandran and Sandra Blakeslee. Good for understanding the strange perceptions that others may have.

Some useful scientific references/books that add more detail.

Books
CRPS for health professionals- a sister volume to this book
Blake in preparation (references fully this text as well). Avalable 2006 Autumn

Complex Regional Pain Syndrome
Harden, Baron, Janig. IASP press

Available from the web including Amazon.
All these books include something on CRPS but are mainly for specialists.

Textbook of pain
Wall, Melzack, (1280 pages)

Neuropathic Pain: From Bench to Bedside
Koltzenburg, Scadding
Psychological Approaches to Pain Management: A Practitioner's Handbook
edited by Turk, Gatchel

A Dictionary of Psychology (Oxford Paperback Reference S.)
Andrew Colman
Pain: A Textbook for Therapists
edited by Strong, Unruh, Wright.

Fibromyalgia & Other Central Pain Syndromes
by Wallance

Pain Management
Edited by Weiner (1138 pages)

Mechanisms and Mediators of Neuropathic Pain
by Malmberg, Chaplan

Pathophysiology of Pain Perception
edited by Lautenbacher, Fillingim

Pain
by Bountra, Munglani, (969 pages)

Hypnosis in the Relief of Pain: Expanding the Goals of Psychotherapy
by Hilgard

A few references and see end of part two for more.

McCabe et al. Rheumatology 2003; 42:1067-1073.

Impaired self-perception
Forderreüther et al. Pain 2004; 110:756-761.
McCabe et al. Pain 2005; 114
3:518-519.

Neglect
Galer et al. J Pain Symptom Manage 1995; 10:385-39
Galer & Jensen. J Pain Symptom Manage 1999; 18:213-217.
Lewis et al. Rheumatology 2003; 42(1):22.

Hemisensory Impairment
Rommel et al. Pain 1999;
80:95-101

Imagined movement
Moseley. Neurology 2004, 62(12):2182-2186.
Schwoebel et al. Brain 2001; 124:2098-2104
McCabe et al. Rheumatology 2003; 42:1067-1073.

And now a scientific review

Part 2

A review of the scientific CRPS literature; conducted 2006

Introduction

THIS REVIEW COVERS WHAT IS PRESENTLY KNOWN ABOUT COMPLEX REGIONAL PAIN SYNDROME (CRPS) AND WHAT IS CURRENT SPECULATION. THE FIRST SECTION EXAMINES HOW THE CLASSIFICATION OF CRPS HAS DEVELOPED INTO THE CURRENTLY ACCEPTED CRITERIA AND THE LIMITATION AND SUGGESTIONS FOR REVISION OF THAT CLASSIFICATION. THE SECOND SECTION DESCRIBES THE VARIED AND COMPLEX SYMPTOMS AND SIGNS THAT FORM THE CLINICAL PRESENTATION. THIRDLY, CURRENT DATA IS PRESENTED ON HOW WIDESPREAD THE CONDITION IS. FINALLY, A REVIEW OF THE CURRENT TREATMENTS AND THEIR LIMITATIONS ARE DISCUSSED.

Why is CRPS important?

CRPS is a painful, debilitating condition, which is poorly understood. The condition greatly affects the individual's ability to function and therefore their quality of life(1). Importantly, the condition is difficult to treat and more than a third deteriorate very seriously over time, experiencing often life long pain and disability as a consequence (2). Although uncommon, the condition is important because it has an array of fascinatingly complex signs and symptoms that present in varied ways and can change over time(3). There is no diagnostic test and diagnosis is made on clinical presentation (4). Given the broad spectrum of symptomatology, patients are often referred to a variety of specialists before a correct diagnosis is made (1). An accurate, timely diagnosis is dependent on the clinician's expertise and the presentation of relevant symptoms that in many cases are not all present at any one time(5).

Often there is a prolonged time period before a confirmed diagnosis is reached(1) causing a sense of frustration to the patient and health professionals in addition to a disproportionate use of healthcare resources(1). Further research is required to better understand CRPS and help address some of these issues.

Classification and diagnostic issues

Classification of CRPS has evolved over time the origins of which were first described by Silas Weir-Mitchell in 1872. He was struck by the presentation of the limbs of soldiers that had sustained a major nerve injury as a consequence of gunshot during the American civil war. Observations of glossy skin, colour changes, burning pain and hyperaesthesia that developed in the distal extremity, spreading beyond the territory of innervation were noted. Mitchell (2) retrospectively termed the phenomena causalgia. Paul Sudeck (6;7) later noted that similar symptoms developed in the limb following a distal bone fracture despite no nerve involvement and termed it Sudeck's atrophy.

More recently, the condition has been known by a variety of different terms. We illustrate a selection of these terms found in the literature. Some terms were introduced in an attempt to reflect the possible mechanisms thought to be responsible for the condition. However the terms are often unclear and confusing. Despite the classification of CRPS being approved a decade ago, a variety of these terms continue to be used both by clinicians and researchers today (8), which adds to the confusion.

The most commonly used alternative term, reflex sympathetic dystrophy (RSD), originally defined disorders that were thought to involve sympathetic nervous system hyperactivity and that responded well to sympathetic nerve blocks (9). However, increasing evidence suggested that a proportion of patients did not respond to sympathetic nerve blocks and no abnormalities in sympathetic nervous system outputs were seen (9). As little was known about the pathology of this condition, the International Association of the Study of Pain (IASP) felt that the term RSD was confusing and potentially misleading.

Former terms were unsatisfactory in adequately describing the condition (9) therefore, the need for a revised taxonomy was felt to be necessary. In November 1993 an IASP working party comprising expert clinicians met in Florida, USA. The outcome of the meeting was the current IASP diagnostic criteria insert (Table 1.)

- Sympathetic dystrophy
- Causalgia
- Algodystrophy
- Sudeck's atrophy
- Algoneurodystrophy
- Painful post traumatic dystrophy
- Shoulder hand syndrome
- Disuse dystrophy
- Traumatic vasospasm
- Post traumatic pain syndrome
- Peripheral acute troponeurosis
- Migratory osteolysis
- Painful post traumatic osteoporosis

*Adapted from McBride and Atkins 2005

The overarching term, complex regional pain syndrome (CRPS) defines a group of painful conditions. *Complex* describes the varied clinical phenomena besides pain; *regional* expresses the distribution of symptoms and signs that are widespread and beyond the area of the original lesion; *pain* is the principal symptom of this group. Subtypes of CRPS, type I and II are classified by the apparent cause and clinical presentation insert (See Table 1.) Type I, formerly known as reflex sympathetic dystrophy (RSD), has no discernable nerve lesion in contrast to type II (formerly causalgia) which has.

Table 1 IASP CRPS classification (Stanton-Hicks et al. 1995)

Complex regional pain syndrome classification criteria (9)	
CRPS Type I	1. Develops after an initiating noxious event 2. Spontaneous pain or allodynia/hyperalgesia occurs, is not limited to the territory of a single peripheral nerve and is disproportionate to the inciting event 3. There is or has been evidence of oedema, skin blood flow abnormality, or abnormal sudomotor activity in the region of the pain since the inciting event. 4. This diagnosis is excluded by the existence of conditions that would otherwise account for the degree of pain and dysfunction
CRPS Type II	1. Develops after a nerve injury. Spontaneous pain or allodynia/hyperalgesia occurs and is not necessarily limited to the territory of the injured nerve. 2. There is or has been evidence of oedema, skin blood flow abnormality, or abnormal sudomotor activity in the region of the pain since the inciting event. 3. This diagnosis is excluded by the existence of conditions that would otherwise account for the degree of pain and dysfunction.

There is dissatisfaction with the current criteria some consider that although the criteria provide standardization for clinical purposes they were consensus derived and lack validation (10). Harden and Bruehl (11) suggest that a consequence of these criteria may be an over or under diagnosis of the syndrome and therefore treatment might be untimely and inappropriate. A factor analysis process of diagnostic and associated signs and symptoms of CRPS, in addition to internal and external validation and a further consensus in Budapest, Hungary in 2003 aimed to improve the criteria.

Two versions of the criteria have been proposed. The first a clinical criteria, is aimed at maximising diagnostic sensitivity, with adequate specificity i.e. sufficiently identifying the condition whilst reducing the effect of over diagnosis and the second a research criteria, aims to balance optimal sensitivity and specificity. Table 2 proposed changes to IASP diagnostic criteria (11)

General definition of the syndrome
CRPS describes an array of painful conditions that are characterised by a continuing (spontaneous and /or evoked) regional pain that is seemingly disproportionate in time or degree to the usual course of any known trauma or other lesion. The pain is regional (not specific nerve territory or dermatome) and usually has a distal predominance of abnormal sensory, motor, sudomotor, vasomotor, and/or trophic findings. The syndrome shows variable progression over time.

| Clinical diagnostic criteria for CRPS | 1. Continued pain disproportionate to any inciting event
2. Must report at least one symptom in three of the four following categories;
    • Sensory: Reports of hyperesthesia and/or allodynia
    • Vasomotor: Reports of temperature asymmetry and/or skin colour changes and /or skin colour asymmetry
    • Sudomotor/oedema; Reports of oedema and/or sweating changes and/or sweating asymmetry.
    • Motor/Trophic: Reports of decreased range of motion and/or motor dysfunction (weakness ,tremor, dystonia) and/or trophic changes(hair ,skin, nails)
4. Must display at least one sign (only counted if observed at time of diagnosis) at time of evaluation in two or more of the following categories:
    • Sensory: Evidence of hyperalgesia (to pinprick) and/or allodynia (to light |

	touch and/or deep somatic pressure and/or joint movement) • Vasomotor: Evidence of temperature asymmetry and/or skin colour changes and /or skin colour asymmetry • Sudomotor/oedema; Evidence of oedema and/or sweating changes and/or sweating asymmetry • Motor/Trophic: Evidence of decreased range of motion and/or motor dysfunction (weakness, tremor, dystonia) and/or trophic changes (hair, skin, nails) 4. There is no other diagnosis that better explains the signs and symptoms
Research diagnostic criteria for CRPS	1. Continued pain disproportionate to any inciting event 2. Must report at least one symptom in each of the four of the symptom categories as above 3. Must display at least one sign (only counted if observed at time of diagnosis) at time of evaluation in two or more of the sign categories described above 4. There is no other diagnosis that better explains the signs and symptoms

Motor and trophic signs and symptoms were added as a subgroup in the criteria as they have been described as important clinical features of the syndrome (1;5).

Of the nature in which these diagnostic criteria have evolved suggests that it has been very difficult to encapsulate exactly what the spectrum of disorders CRPS represents, in a single diagnostic framework. Furthermore, the complex nature of this procedure illustrates the difficulty in diagnosing this condition. Although the proposed new, rather lengthy, definition goes some way to improve validity (11), further work is required in order to establish sound workable criteria suitable for both clinical and research purposes.

Diagnostic issues have been well documented(2;8;12). In a retrospective study of 134 cases that attended a chronic pain clinic in the USA, the mean duration between symptom onset and attending the specialist unit was 2.5 years(1). The authors suggest that one of the main difficulties was the lack of ability to identify the condition amongst primary care physicians. Furthermore, the study highlights the excessive number of specialists (Mean 4.8) the patient visits prior to attending an appropriate specialist unit. This has implications on healthcare resources and possibly delays the commencement of appropriate treatment intervention. Limitations of the study are that it was based on data derived from case notes with no standardised systematic data collection method and from one clinic. Although this is an American study and therefore may not be representative of the UK, the findings raise some important issues that merit further investigation, particularly in the UK where no such data is published.

The lack of a timely, clear diagnosis coupled with the distress of symptoms can have an emotional impact on patients causing fear, anxiety and depression (2). Studies exploring these issues were few. There was a recent prospective study investigating depression in those following a distal radial fracture who then developed CRPS(13). Individuals were being monitored for the development of signs of the diagnosis therefore it was identified very rapidly at two months post fracture and depression levels were not significantly different from those that did not develop CRPS. Hence patients did not experience a prolonged period of visiting other specialists before eventually receiving a diagnosis that is likely to contribute towards a depressive state. These issues merit further research.

Clinical features of CRPS

CRPS is characterised by various signs and symptoms as described below. The severity of the symptoms is disproportionate to the severity of the inciting trauma and are not necessarily limited to the dermatome of the affected nerve (14). Typically not all signs and symptoms may be present at any one time making diagnosis difficult (2). Furthermore, the patient symptom report is crucial in the diagnostic assessment.

Pain

Pain, the cardinal symptom, is described by patients as deep, shooting, throbbing and burning (2;5;9) which exceeds the normal tissue healing time and is disproportionate to the inciting event(9). Pain extends often distally beyond the site of the initial trauma and has no spatial relation to nerve territories (3). Spontaneous, and more clinically striking, is the presentation of stimulus evoked pains (14). Mechanical and or thermal allodynia and hyperalgesia are often so severe that contact with, or active movement by, the affected part is avoided and the patient often exhibits guarding behaviour to protect the affected limb (2). Patients report extreme sensitivity to temperature changes such as air draught and when bathing (5). Janig and Baron (3) recently observed that stimulus evoked pain is typically produced by deep somatic tissue as a consequence of movements and pressure at the joints which bear no relation to the initial trauma site. Five percent of patients presented with stimulus evoked pain only rather than spontaneous pain (3). However, Veldman (8) reported that 7% of 829 patients studied prospectively, presented with neither spontaneous or stimulus evoked pain yet met the diagnostic criteria for RSD.

Sudomotor changes

Abnormal sweating patterns are characteristic. Studies suggest that excessive sweating (hyperhidrosis) is more common in the early stages. Velman (8) reported that 57% of acute CRPS cases presented with hyperhidrosis, although Wasner(14) reported excessive sweating in both acute and chronic stages. Hypohidrosis (subnormal sweating) is less common (14) and seen in the later stages. Interestingly, unilateral sweating abnormalities present in the affected limb only have been noted (14).

Vasomotor changes

Changes in skin temperature and blood flow are apparent. Studies gave varying reports of the prevalence of temperature changes. Veldman et al (8) found that 86% of their sample presented with either warmer or colder affected limbs. Wasner et al (14) suggested as little as 30% have a measurably hotter or colder limb when compared to the unaffected side in a constant room temperature controlled environment. The limb is often

213

warmer in the early stages and as the disease progresses (greater than 6 months) skin temperature and blood flow decrease (14). Furthermore, Janig and Baron(3) found that in the acute stages, induced body cooling and respiratory stimuli did not trigger the normal response of vasoconstriction.

Colour asymmetry of the affected limb changes to mottled, red and purple (5). Oedema is often present in the acute stages and extends well beyond the region of the inciting trauma (2;3;8).

Trophic changes

Studies report that an abnormal growth pattern of hair and nails is a further feature of the condition (2;8;14). In Veldman's study (8) 55% and 60% of cases had growth abnormalities of the hair and nails respectively. These changes happen only on the affected limb where nails often grow excessively and are thickened. Skin hair becomes thick, dark and coarse. Skin texture changes to become thin and glossy or thickened (14). Nodular fasciitis was evident in 20% of Veldman's sample (8). Trophic changes can appear within weeks of onset (15).

Motor/functional changes

Motor changes are reported in the literature in varying prevalence and to varying degrees. Janig et al. (3) suggest that 70% present with muscle weakness of the affected limb whilst Veldman et al. (1993) report the prevalence is much greater (95%). Similarly, active range of motion is reduced as soft tissue contractures limit movement and consequently cause loss of function (9), particularly in small accurate movements (3). Interestingly, nerve conduction studies are normal suggestive of a normal peripheral motor system (3). Both Veldman et al. (1993) and Janig and Baron (2003) suggest that about half experience a tremor of the affected limb and 54% present with uncoordinated movements. Dystonia of the affected extremity is less common (10%) (3;14). Furthermore, muscle spasm was a feature in 25% of chronic cases (8). Exercise exacerbates the symptoms and Veldman et al (8) reported that 121 out of 829 patients were unable to actively move their affected limb. Pain protection behaviour is a causal factor.

Body perception disturbance

Galer et al(16;17) Forderreuther(18) and Moseley (19) have all found evidence suggestive of changes in body perception. These have been documented but will be discussed at length in the following section.

Psychological factors

Psychological distress symptoms have been widely acknowledged as being a feature of CRPS. Although there has been debate as to whether this is a cause or consequence. Earlier studies reporting distress symptoms coupled with normal neuro physiological results suggested that CRPS was principally psychogenic. More recently however, the view is that this distress is a reaction to and therefore a consequence of the persistent and severe symptoms of CRPS (2;14). No studies were found within the literature that explored these issues qualitatively in a methodologically sound manner. Moreover, there were no qualitative studies regarding the subjective experience of any aspect of adult complex regional pain syndrome. There is a clear need to develop research in this area.

How common is CRPS?

Little data assessing the epidemiology of this condition has been published which is due in the main, to the complexity of the diagnostic criteria therefore knowledge regarding incidence and the course of the condition is restricted (2). Current epidemiological studies have all been undertaken in countries other than the UK. Furthermore, despite retrospective studies (1), very few prospective studies have been undertaken(8;12). However, Sandroni et al. (12) undertook a retrospective population based study of 106,470 people in Minnesota. Using IASP criteria for CRPS type I they reported an incidence rate of 5.57 per 100,000 person years at risk and a period prevalence of 20.7 per 100,000.

Current evidence suggests that between two to four times more women develop CRPS than men (2.3:1(1;1) 3:1 (8) and 4:1(12) respectively). The median age at symptom onset is between 37.7 years (1) and 46 years (12).

The ethic origin of those studied was predominantly Caucasian (1;12). This finding must be interpreted with caution as where data was available; the populations studied were up to 80% Caucasian.

Precipitating events

A variety of precipitating events are documented in the literature of which trauma is the most common accounting for up to 65% of cases (8). Fracture is the principal traumatic cause and there is evidence to suggest that up to 37% develop CRPS following distal radial fractures(20). Other invasive interventions such as injections, intravenous infusions and surgery were also reported as triggers (1;2;8;12). Furthermore, disease processes such as stroke and myocardial ischemia were noted as precipitating events. Interestingly there were a number of recorded cases (10% Veldman et al. (1995)) where no identifiable preceding event was identified. It could be speculated that the disease spontaneously occurred whilst others suggest that the trauma may be too small to be discernable. However, why do most people that suffer trauma not go on to develop CRPS? There is evolving evidence to suggest that genetic factors may have an influence. Van Hilten (21) found significantly raised HLA-DR13 in a sample of CRPS presenting with dystonia when compared with controls. However, the sample of 26 was small so further research is required to qualify these preliminary findings.

Disease presentation and progression

The upper limb is more commonly affected than the lower limb (4;12). Veldman et al. (1995) reported upper limb involvement at one and a half times that of the lower limb although these findings don't appear to account for the possible spread of the condition.

Despite the condition starting in one limb there is evidence that it spreads not only to other limbs but also to other body parts. Veldman et al. (8;12)reported that more than one limb was affected in 39 out of 615 of those with CRPS type I. Data further showed that four patients had involvement of three limbs and one patient had CRPS type I of all limbs. Bladder and bowels have also reportedly been involved(22). It is unclear from the evidence however whether this is just related to lower limb CRPS (23)

216

There is little data on the long term outcomes in CRPS. According to Sandroni et al. (2003), seventy four percent of cases resolved often spontaneously. However, clinical experience suggests that a proportion go on to develop severely disabling disease for up to twenty years later. CRPS has a negative impact on work and relationships(2).

Treatment

The aims of treatment are to provide pain relief and achieve functional restoration (5;11;15). Given the difficulties in diagnosis in particular, the prolonged time period to achieve an accurate one, appropriate treatment in often delayed(1).

Medication

Pharmaceutical interventions are numerous. Although there are few randomised controlled trials little evidence regarding drug efficacy in CRPS exists thus current practice is based on a trial and error approach (15). A brief overview of medication will be given.

Non-steroidal anti inflammatories (NSAIDS) such as diclofenac and celecoxib are used for pain relief and to reduce inflammation(15). Opioids such as codeine, morphine and tramadol are a more potent option which are used with caution given their addictive properties(15) Analgesics acting on central mechanisms are also prescribed. These include anti epileptics such as gabapentin and pregabalin and anti depressants such as amitripyline. Bisphosphanates such as pamidronate and calcitonin are used for pain and bone regeneration. Topical treatments such as capsaicin can also be used.

Other therapeutic interventions

As a key treatment objective in CRPS is that of functional restoration, Occupational Therapists and Physiotherapists play a major role within the multidisciplinary team. There is very little evidence to prove the efficacy of specific treatment techniques. Furthermore, in the majority of articles where treatment techniques have been mentioned, there is no supporting evidence or in some cases detail about how to implement the technique(5;11;15). Studies that have been undertaken are on small numbers so can be regarded as preliminary at this stage (24;25).

In addition to the paucity of evidence, the CRPS patient may present with a broad array of signs and symptoms at any one time that fluctuate in intensity and duration. Therefore, the therapist has to undertake a thorough assessment and implement treatment options generally on a trial and error basis. Mobilisation techniques include active stretching and gradual gentle movements which are undertaken within the patients tolerance (5). One study has suggested that active pressure on the limbs can also be applied through the technique of stress loading (26) although clinical experience is that patients often cannot or do not wish to get down and support themselves on the ground on all four limbs as the programme suggests.

Desensitisation techniques consist of giving tactile sensory inputs. These are provided by a variety of textures such as cotton wool and silk to assist in normalising sensory responses. This technique is mentioned in a number of studies but no detail is given regarding the strategy i.e. intensity and duration of the activities and exact materials used. (5; 11; 15).

Other more novel techniques include mirror visual feedback (MVF), which involves the use of a mirror placed between the limbs such that the affected limb is hidden behind and the unaffected limb is reflected in the mirror. The patient views the reflection of the unaffected limb as if it was the affected limb. The mode of action is thought to be that visual feedback will influence the normalisation of cortical processing. McCabe et al. (27) piloted MVF on eight CRPS type I patients with up to three years duration. Results showed that the technique was affective in reducing pain and sudomotor changes in those with disease duration of less than a year but not the chronic cases. Moseley (25) combined MVF with graded imagery techniques which involved asking the patients to imagine carrying out the movement pictured on a card with their affected hand. Those with chronic CRPS type I showed better pain and swelling reduction than those undertaking MVF alone. As previously mentioned these are preliminary studies that require further investigation on a larger study population.

The literature strongly supports the need for interventions to be implemented as early as possible to ensure better outcomes (4;5;11;28).However, given the difficulties in obtaining an accurate diagnosis, early treatment intervention is often not achieved (1).

BODY PERCEPTION AND RELATED DISTURBANCES

This section describes what is understood by the term body perception. We then discuss relevant examples of conditions with an associated disruption in body perception. Current literature pertaining to body perception disturbance in CRPS is examined and the limitation of existing knowledge is discussed.

What is body perception?

Body perception can be described, in short, as the cortical representation of the body. There are a variety of representations of the body within the brain (29;30). Firstly, there is the awareness of the body at a conscious cognitive level which is termed as body image (29;30). Body image occurs consciously, whereby visual body representation relates to how one sees one's body as well as conceptual knowledge about the body (29). Coslett (31) describes it as 'the way the body appears from the outside' and is associated with a semantic representation. Pathologies of body image include anorexia and bulimia(32).

Body schema on the other hand, is the cortical representation of the body responsible for the spatial organisation of action and typically occurs at the unconscious level (29). This is an important distinction that should be drawn between body schema and body image. There is little evidence to suggest that body image influences body schema (Haggard et al 2004). Therefore, pure disorders of body image are considered to be not relevant to this work and shall not be discussed. However there are cases where body schema affects body image which will be described further on in this chapter.

Head and Holmes (33) gave one of the earliest accounts of body perception and introduced the term 'body schema'. This concept, prompted by patient observations of cases with a parietal cortex lesion, was described by Head and Holmes as a disordered spatial representation of the body. They proposed a 'postural model of ourselves that is always changing' (pg 187) is represented in the brain. Furthermore, they hypothesised that somatosensory and proprioceptive

219

inputs generated a constantly changing 'postural model' of one's body. When limbs are no longer moving there is no sensory information to update the body schema.

The concept of body schema as suggested by Head and Holmes, hypothesized that the body schema is passively updated which is an unconscious process. Furthermore, that the updating was due to somatosensory and proprioceptive inputs alone. Move recent work in this area provides evidence that this is not always the case.

Body schema processes are behind what appears to be a simple coordinated and controlled action such that a complex interaction of proprioceptive, vestibular, somatosensory and visual inputs interrelates with motor systems. In order to produce these seemingly effortless movements of the body through space, the brain must constantly monitor the position and movement of the body in relation to nearby objects and in order to be able to pick them up (29). Unconscious cognitive judgements about the weight of a cup, for example, the effort required in picking it up and knowledge of body parts and their relationship to each other are made in order to execute the action accurately. The process of multimodal sensory integration forms an on-line neural representational map of the body that is stored in the cortex(34). This representation is constantly updated through experience of repeated patterns of movements. Inputs are not just restricted to proprioceptive and somatosensory modalities alone as Head and Holmes hypothesised, more recent evidence suggests that visual inputs are also influential(29;35;36).

A further cortical body representation is that of a somatosensory nature. It is well known that inputs from sensory skin and proprioceptive receptors project contra laterally to a topographical map within the cortex known as the Penfield Homunculus (37). This sensory homunculus is located within the primary somatosensory cortex, SI. This we illustrated in part 1.
The cortical representation of the body within the homunculus is not anatomically correct such that the head is next to the hand and the feet adjacent to the genitalia. Furthermore, particular areas of the body such as the lips, hands and genitalia are over sized, depicting greater representation than other areas such as the back. This can be explained as these areas have a greater density of sensory receptors within the skin enabling extreme sensitivity to touch and fine discrimination (38).

220

Body perception disorders

So far, evidence to suggest that the body is cortically represented in a variety of ways has been discussed. Aspects of how disorders can influence body perception will be examined to help further our understanding.

Phantom limb is a common phenomena in amputees(38;39). The phenomenon is described as when an amputee still experiences sensations of the missing limb. Such sensations are typically that of movement, pain and stiffness (38;40;41)

Recent studies have shown that sensations of the amputated limb are felt when another part of the intact body is touched. Ramachandran (38) demonstrated that a patient with an amputated arm felt parts of the hand being touched when his face was stroked. The amputee was blindfolded to prevent any influence from visual input. These were localised sensations within a topographical area such that specific parts of the hand could be precisely mapped out on the face. Further findings suggest that these referred sensations are modality specific i.e. if a cold object touches the faces then a cold sensation is elicited from the phantom. Evidence is provided to suggest that as neurons responsible for the amputated area are no longer receiving any sensory input, then adjacent neurons representing other body parts invade the area, activating the denervated area as well as their own(39). This demonstrates that cortical reorganisation or neuro plasticity within the somatosensory homunculus has taken place.

Evidence of body perception disturbance in CRPS

Recent studies have suggested that pain has an influence on cortical body representation.

Schwoebel (42) showed pictures of right and left hands in various positions to thirteen subjects with unilateral upper limb CRPS and eighteen aged matched controls. The participants were asked to state whether a right or left hand was pictured and reaction times were recorded. This task involved mentally rotating ones hand, supporting evidence that it concerns the body schema. When reaction times of the affected limb were compared to those of the unaffected upper limb for large amplitude movements they were greater than matched controls. This would suggest that pain has an influence on disturbing the body scheme. A small sample size was a limiting factor of this study.

Other studies have produced evidence to support the theory that the cortical representation of the body is disrupted in CRPS. McCabe et al. (43) repeated Ramachandrans (38) referred sensations experiment on a small sample of CRPS I participants. She found similar findings in that five out of sixteen participants reported somatosensory feelings elicited from a body part other than, but in association with, the area being stimulated with their eyes closed. Stimulation of the hand elicited somatosensations of the ipsilateral cheek. Likewise stimulation of the sole of the foot elicited feelings below the ipsilateral knee in one participant but occurred in reverse in another. These sensations were modality specific and diminished or were no longer present when the body was viewed. These referred sensations can perhaps only partly be explained by neural changes within the sensory homunculus as topographically, the face is adjacent to the hand, but the foot is not next to the knee. However, these findings are particularly interesting as there is no known peripheral denervation within CRPS I. Why this occurs is currently unknown.

Brain imaging has enabled a deeper understanding of cortical body representation in CRPS. Juottonen (44) used magneto encephalography (MEG) to examine six right handed patients with unilateral upper limb CRPS. Cortical responses to tactile stimuli of individual digits of both hands were recorded in both hemispheres. Responses in the contra lateral S1 hemisphere demonstrated that the cortical representation of the thumb to little finger of the affected hand had reduced by up to 40 percent when compared to the contra lateral cortical map of the unaffected digits. This provides evidence of shrinkage in cortical representation of the CRPS hand. There was no evidence of a correlation between degree of shrinkage and intensity or duration of pain. This study is limited by a small, all female sample with symptom duration of 1 to 6 years therefore not representative of the general CRPS population. However it does add weight to the evidence for cortical neuroplasticity in CRPS.

A more recent study by Maihofner (45) undertook a longitudinal study on the cortical mapping within S1 of those with unilateral upper limb CRPS. Using MEG and MRI the baseline scans were taken between 4 and 36 weeks after initial symptom onset. Follow up scans were undertaken at a mean time of 58 weeks later. Results showed that the distance taken mid first to fifth digit and that of the lip had increased at follow up when compared to baseline measures. Comparing the follow up cortical measurement of the affected side to that of the unaffected side the distance had not returned to normal. All participants reported reduced pain scores on the McGill pain questionnaire at follow up. These scores correlated with the enlarged cortical distance and Maihofner el al. have suggested that there is a correlation between a reduction in pain and a return to the normal cortical spacing of affected body parts within S1. Maihofner further argues that this normalisation is due to therapy but there was no explanation as to the specific interventions, intensity, dose or duration of therapy. It could be argued that spontaneous recovery was responsible for the reduction in symptoms and a return to a normal cortical map. It would be interesting to see what changes happen cortically when pain persists or increases over time.

Clinical presentations of body perception disturbance in CRPS

The first documented descriptions of the phenomenon explored in this study, were presented by Galer et al. (46;47). In the first of two papers(48) they presented eleven case studies that described a motor dysfunction and feelings of the affected limb being 'disconnected' from consciousness. Motor dysfunction was not clearly defined but included patient reports that the affected limb was difficult to move and clinical observations that movement initiation was belated, there were fewer spontaneous movements and the amplitude of movement was reduced. The cases were selected by the authors from their clinical caseload of patients diagnosed with CRPS type I spanning a period of 22 months. No defined inclusion or exclusion criteria were given. Although it was reported that a neglect battery was used for selection, it was not stated what this comprised. There was no methodological detail about how the patients' descriptions were captured.

Galer et al. hypothesised that the clinical presentations were similar to neurological neglect and therefore termed the phenomenon a neglect-like disorder. Furthermore, it was suggested that nine out of 11 participants described a form similar to asomatoagnosia or the denial of

223

a body part again it was not ascertained as to how this conclusion was drawn.

The second paper (49), introduced the notion of cognitive neglect. In addition to motor neglect. This was defined as patients that perceived that their affected limb was not part of their being. How the theory of cognitive neglect had developed from the first paper was not discussed. In particular, there was no mention of asomatoagnosia.

Based on these two aspects of motor and cognitive neglect, the aim of the second study was to determine the frequency of neglect symptoms in CRPS. A two part questionnaire was posted to members of a national reflex sympathetic dystrophy (RSD now termed CRPS I) syndrome society. The first section of the questionnaire comprised patient demographics, symptomology and duration of symptoms. The second part comprised five statements devised by Galer based on clinical experience. Two statements were intended to represent cognitive neglect and two, motor neglect. The fifth statement was not relevant to either. Respondents were asked to tick any statement that applied to them.

The first section of the questionnaire was evaluated by one of the researchers to ascertain a diagnosis of CRPS I. In the second section it was determined that if one or more of the four neglect statements was ticked then the respondent had neglect like symptoms.
Results suggested that of the 242 respondents, 232 were confirmed with CRPS I and of those 84% had neglect like symptoms of which 47% had both motor and cognitive neglect.

There were a number of flaws in this study. Firstly, it could be suggested that there is an element of bias. The group were self-selecting and the questionnaire self administered therefore there was no objective clinical assessment to ascertain diagnosis or signs of motor neglect. The diagnosis based on information given on the questionnaire was ascertained by one of the researchers and not an independent assessor therefore the results could be susceptible to bias. The statements were devised by the researcher based on his experience alone therefore may not reflect all aspects of their theory.

No information was given on piloting the statements to ensure firstly, that they accurately reflected the nature of the symptoms, secondly that they

224

did not have more than one meaning and finally, that they were not leading.

In light of the flawed methodology the findings should be interpreted with caution.

Interestingly though, Galer et al. (50;51) theorised that these neglect like symptoms were due to a dysfunction in the motor and orientation systems within the CNS rather than any disturbance in the body schema.

More recent studies such as Forderreuther and Moseley (52-54) present further findings that allude more to a body perception disorder rather than a neglect-like syndrome.

Forderreuther et al. (55) asked 73 participants with upper limb CRPS to name the fingers touched with a cotton swab both on the affected and unaffected side. Forty eight percent were unable to identify one or more fingers on their affected hand and 6.5% fingers on their unaffected had. Further more, participants were asked what feeling they had towards their affected hand followed up with prompts such as 'foreign' or 'strange'. Fifty four percent were reported to have expressed these feelings. In addition to this, participants were also tested for hemi spatial neglect using the line bisection and sensory distinction tests. These results were normal.

It was unclear from the method whether the participants viewed their fingers in the test. Furthermore, given the bias prompts it could be suggested that the way in which information was gained regarding how the hands felt, was leading. Forderreuther concluded that these findings were not classic neglect but an impairment of self-perception suggestive of cortical reorganisation.

Moseley adds weight to this argument(54). By showing a series of increasingly enlarged pictures of the CRPS participants' hands and comparing the selected picture to the actual measurement of the hand, he reported that participants chose a pictured hand a mean of 3% larger than the size of their actual hand.

He suggested that this distortion in body image was due to cortical reorganisation indicative of changes in S1 and visual systems.

What is known is that patients report a strangeness of their affected hands that is not part of their body although these data has not been collected in a systematically methodologically sound manner.

225

Observations have shown that they also visually perceive their affected hand as larger than they are, have impaired finger identification and have difficulty in initiating and co-ordinating movements.

Yet no one has asked those with CRPS to describe their affected limbs. Subjective data has not been systematically collected on how those with CRPS perceive their affected limbs.

Further research is required to address these aspects by undertaking a qualitative approach to explore the experience of body perception disturbance in CRPS.

Reference List

(1) Allen G, Galer BS, Schwartz L. Epidemiology of complex regional pain syndrome: a retrospective chart review of 134 patients. Pain 1999;80(3):539-44.

(2) Scadding JW. Complex regional pain syndrome. In: Wall PD, Melzack R, editors. Textbook of Pain. 4th ed. Edinburgh: Churchill Livingston; 1999. p. 835-49.

(3) Janig W, Baron R. Complex Regional Pain Syndrome: mystery explained? The Lancet Neurology 2003;30:687-97.

(4) McBride A, Atkins R. Complex regional pain syndrome. Current Orthopaedics 2005;. 19(2).

(5) Harden RN. Complex Regional Pain Syndrome. British Journal of Anaesthesia 2001;87(1):99-106.

(6) Sudeck P. Uber die acute entzundliche knochenatrophie. Arch Klin Chir 1900;62:147-56.

(7) Sudeck P. Die sogen. Akute knochenatrophie als entzundungsvorgang. Der Chirurg 1942;15:449-58.   (8) Veldman P, Reynen H, Arntz I, Goris R. Signs and symptoms of reflex sympathetic dystrophy: prospective study of 829 patients. The Lancet 1993;342:1012-6.

(9) Stanton-Hicks M, Janig W, Hassenbusch S, Haddox JD, Boas R, Wilson P. Reflex sympathetic dystrophy: Changing concepts and taxonomy. Pain 1995;63:127-33.

(10) Bruehl S, Harden RN, Galer BS, Saltz S, Bertram M, Backonja M, et al. External validation of IASP diagnostic criteria for complex regional pain syndrome and proposed research diagnostic criteria. Pain 1999 May;81(1-2):147-54.

(11) Wilson P, Stanton-Hicks M, Harden RN. CRPS: Current diagnosis and therapy. Seattle: IASP Press; 2005.

(12) Sandroni P, Benrud-Larson L, McClelland R, Low P. Complex regional pain syndrome type I:incidence and prevalence in Olmsted county, a population-based study. Pain 2003;103(1-2):199-207.

(13) Puchalski P, Zyluk A. Complex regional pain syndrome type 1 after fractures of the distal radius: A prospective study of the role of psychological factors. Journal of Hand Surgery-British and European Volume 2005;30B(6):574-80.

(14) Wasner G, Schattschneider J, Binder A, Baron R. Complex regional pain syndrome - diagnostic, mechanisms, CNS involvement and therapy. Spinal Cord 2003;41:61-75.

(15) Stanton-Hicks M, Baron R, Boas R, Gordh T, Harden RN, Hendler N, et al. Complex regional pain syndromes: Guidelines for therapy. The Clinical Journal of Pain 1998;14:155-66.

(16) Galer BS, Jensen M. Neglect-like symptoms in complex regional pain syndrome: results of a self-administered survey 3. J Pain Symptom Manage 1999 Sep;18(3):213-7.

(17) Galer BS, Butler S, Jensen MP. Case reports and hypothesis: a neglect-like syndrome may be responsible for the motor disturbance in reflex sympathetic dystrophy (Complex Regional Pain Syndrome-1). J Pain Symptom Manage 1995 Jul;10(5):385-91.

(18) Forderreuther S, Sailer U, Straube A. Impaired self-perception of the hand in complex regional pain syndrome (CRPS) 1. Pain 2004 Aug;110(3):756-61.

(19) Moseley GL. Why do people with complex regional pain syndrome take longer to recognize their affected hand? Neurology 2004 Jun 22;62(12):2182-6.

(20) Atkins RM, Duckworth T, Kanis J. Features of algodystrophy following Colles fracture. Journal of Bone and Joint Surgery 1990;72B:105-10.

(21) van Hilten JJ, van de Beek WJ, Roep BO, van Hilten JJ, van de Beek WJ, Roep BO. Multifocal or generalized tonic dystonia of complex regional pain syndrome: a distinct clinical entity associated with HLA-DR13. Annals of Neurology 2000 Jul;48(1):113-6.

(22) van Hilten JJ, van de Beek WJT, Roep BO. Multifocal or generalized tonic dystonia of complex regional pain syndrome: A distinct clinical entity associated with HLA-DR13. Annals of Neurology 2000 Jul;48(1):113-6.

(23) Galloway NT, Gabale DR, Irwin PP, Galloway NT, Gabale DR, Irwin PP. Interstitial cystitis or reflex sympathetic dystrophy of the bladder? Seminars in Urology 1991 May;9(2):148-53.

(24) McCabe CS, Haigh RC, Ring EFJ, Halligan PW, Wall PD, Blake DR. A controlled pilot study of the utility of mirror visual feedback in the treatment of complex regional pain syndrome (type 1). Rheumatology 2003 Jan;42(1):97-101.

(25) Moseley GL. Graded motor imagery is effective for long-standing complex regional pain syndrome: a randomised controlled trial. Pain 2004;108(1-2):192-8.

(26) Carlson L, Watson H. Treatment of reflex sympathetic dystrophy using the stress loading program. Journal of Hand Therapy 1988;1:149-54.

(27) McCabe CS, Haigh RC, Ring EFJ, Halligan PW, Wall PD, Blake DR. A controlled pilot study of the utility of mirror visual feedback in the treatment of complex regional pain syndrome (type 1). Rheumatology 2003 Jan;42(1):97-101.

(28) McCabe CS, Haigh RC, Ring EFJ, Halligan PW, Wall PD, Blake DR. A controlled pilot study of the utility of mirror visual feedback in the treatment of complex regional pain syndrome (type 1). Rheumatology 2003 Jan;42(1):97-101.

(29) Haggard P, Wolpert D. Disorders of Body Scheme. Higher-Order Motor Disorders 2005.

(30) Coslett HB. Anosognosia and body representations forty years later. Cortex 2005;41(2):263-70.

(31) Coslett H. Evidence for a disturbance of the body schema in neglect. Brain and Cognition 1998;37:527-44.

(32) Farrell C, Lee M, Shafran R. Assessment of body size estimation: A review. European Eating Disorders Review 2005;13:75-88.

(33) Head H, Holmes G. Sensory disturbances from cerebral lesions. Brain 1911;2(34):102-254.

(34) Haggard P, Taylor-Clarke M, Kennett S. Tactile perception, cortical representation and the bodily self. Current Biology 2003;13(5):R170-R173.

(35) Graziano MSA, Cooke DF, Taylor CSR. Coding the location of the arm by sight. Science 2000 Dec 1;290(5497):1782-6.

(36) Kennett S, Taylor-Clarke M, Haggard P. Noninformative vision improves the spatial resolution of touch in humans. Current Biology 2001;11(15):1188-91.

(37) Penfield W, Rasmussen T. The cerebral cortex of man; a clinical study of localization of function. 1950.

(38) Ramachandran VS. Phantoms in the brain. London: Fourth Estate; 1999.

(39) Ramachandran VS. Plasticity and functional recovery in neurology. Clinical Medicine 2005;5(4):368-73.

(40) Haigh RC, McCabe CS, Halligan PW, Blake DR. Joint stiffness in a phantom limb: evidence of central nervous system involvement in rheumatoid arthritis. Rheumatology (Oxford) 2003 Jul;42(7):888-92.

(41) Fraser CM, Halligan PW, Robertson IH, Kirker SG. Characterising phantom limb phenomena in upper limb amputees. Prosthet Orthot Int 2001 Dec;25(3):235-42.

(42) Schwoebel J, Coslett HB, Bradt J, Friedman R, Dileo C. Pain and the body schema: Effects of pain severity on mental representations of movement. Neurology 2002;59(5):775-7.

(43) McCabe CS, Haigh RC, Halligan PW, Blake DR. Referred sensations in patients with complex regional pain syndrome type 1. Rheumatology (Oxford) 2003 Sep;42(9):1067-73.

(44) Juottonen K, Gockel M, Silen T, Hurri H, Hari R, Forss N. Altered central sensorimotor processing in patients with complex regional pain syndrome. Pain 2002;98(3):315-23.

(45) Maihofner C, Handwerker HO, Neundorfer B, Birklein F. Cortical reorganization during recovery from complex regional pain syndrome. Neurology 2004;63(4):693-701.

(46) Galer BS, Butler S, Jensen MP. Case reports and hypothesis: a neglect-like syndrome may be responsible for the motor disturbance in reflex sympathetic dystrophy (Complex Regional Pain Syndrome-1). J Pain Symptom Manage 1995 Jul;10(5):385-91.

(47) Galer BS, Jensen M. Neglect-like symptoms in complex regional pain syndrome: results of a self-administered survey. J Pain Symptom Manage 1999 Sep;18(3):213-7.

(48) Galer BS, Butler S, Jensen MP. Case reports and hypothesis: a neglect-like syndrome may be responsible for the motor disturbance in reflex sympathetic dystrophy (Complex Regional Pain Syndrome-1). J Pain Symptom Manage 1995 Jul;10(5):385-91.

(49) Galer BS, Jensen M. Neglect-like symptoms in complex regional pain syndrome: results of a self-administered survey. J Pain Symptom Manage 1999 Sep;18(3):213-7.

(50) Galer BS, Jensen M. Neglect-like symptoms in complex regional pain syndrome: results of a self-administered survey. J Pain Symptom Manage 1999 Sep;18(3):213-7.

(51)   Galer BS, Butler S, Jensen MP. Case reports and hypothesis: a neglect-like syndrome may be responsible for the motor disturbance in reflex sympathetic dystrophy (Complex Regional Pain Syndrome-1). J Pain Symptom Manage 1995 Jul;10(5):385-91.

(52)   Forderreuther S, Sailer U, Straube A. Impaired self-perception of the hand in complex regional pain syndrome (CRPS) 1. Pain 2004 Aug;110(3):756-61.

(53)   Moseley GL. Why do people with complex regional pain syndrome take longer to recognize their affected hand? Neurology 2004 Jun 22;62(12):2182-6.

(54)   Moseley L. Distorted body image in complex regional pain syndrome. Neurology 2005;65(1):773.

(55)   Forderreuther S, Sailer U, Straube A. Impaired self-perception of the hand in complex regional pain syndrome (CRPS) 1. Pain 2004 Aug;110(3):756-61.

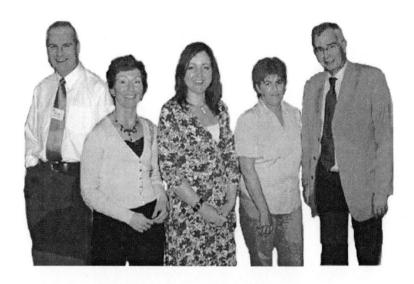

"Spreading the RSD word"

David Blake, Catherine Taylor, Jenny Lewis,
Candy Mc Cabe and Barry Swallow.

Please help us by making a donation to RSD UK

Any profits from this book go to two charities.

RSD UK is a voluntary non-profit making charity which was set up to give support to those concerned with Reflex Sympathetic Dystrophy/Complex Regional Pain Syndrome.

The Bath Institute for Rheumatic Disease (BIRD) is an independent registered charity which raises funds to support research and education into many aspects of bone and joint diseases.